Handbook of Analytical Methods for Dietary Supplements

Handbook of Analytical Methods for Dietary Supplements

Frank Jaksch, Mingfu Wang, and Mark Roman

American Pharmacists Association™
Improving medication use. Advancing patient care.
APhA
Washington, D.C.

Managing Editor: Vicki Meade, Meade Communications
Acquiring Editor: Sandra J. Cannon
Copy Editor: L. Luan Corrigan, Corrigan Editorial Services
Proofreaders: Gurpriya Gill and Mary-Ann Moalli, Publications Professionals LLC
Indexer: Suzanne Peake
Book Layout: Roy Barnhill
Editorial Assistant: Kellie Burton

Published by the American Pharmacists Association
2215 Constitution Ave., NW
Washington, DC 20037-2985
www.aphanet.org

APhA was founded in 1852 as the American Pharmaceutical Association.

To comment on this book via e-mail, send your message to the publisher at aphabooks @aphanet.org.

Library of Congress Cataloging-in-Publication Data

Jaksch, Frank, b. 1968-
Handbook of analytical methods for dietary supplements / Frank Jaksch, Mingfu Wang, and Mark Roman.
p. ; cm.
Includes bibliographical references and index.
ISBN 1-58212-055-2
1. Dietary supplements--Analysis.
[DNLM: 1. Dietary Supplements--analysis--Laboratory Manuals. 2. Plant Preparations--analysis--Laboratory Manuals. 3. Plants, Medicinal--analysis--Laboratory Manuals. QU 25 J25h 2005] I. Wang, Mingfu, b. 1972- II. Roman, Mark, b. 1967- III. American Pharmacists Association. IV. Title.

RM258.5.J34 2005
615'.1--dc22

2005006579

How to Order This Book
Online: www.pharmacist.com
By phone: 800-878-0729
VISA®, MasterCard®, and American Express® cards accepted.

Contents

About the Authors

Frank Jaksch is president, chief executive officer, and cofounder of ChromaDex, Inc., a company in Santa Ana, California, that creates and supplies botanical reference standards and related phytochemical products and services. Jaksch brings to the company leadership and vision, as well as significant technical, sales, and marketing experience in scientific products, pharmaceuticals, and nutraceuticals. He holds a BS in chemistry and biology from Valparaiso University.

Mingfu Wang, PhD, is assistant research professor in the New Use Agriculture and Natural Plant Products Program at Rutgers University. In addition to heading the natural products lab and training scientists, he works to identify novel bioactive compounds and develop analytical protocols for the chemical characterization of aromatic and medicinal plants and functional foods. Wang earned his BS in chemistry from Ocean University of Qingdao, China; MS in organic chemistry from Shanghai Institute of Materia Medica, Chinese Academy of Science; and PhD in food science from Rutgers University.

Mark Roman, PhD, is director of research and development (R&D) at ChromaDex, Inc., overseeing the analytical test method development and validation program as well as day-to-day operations of the ChromaDex R&D laboratory in Clearwater, Florida. Roman, with over 15 years' R&D experience in the chemical, pharmaceutical, and dietary supplement industries, has a BS in chemistry from the University of Delaware, and PhD in analytical chemistry from the University of Rhode Island. He is 2005 chair of the AOAC International Methods Review Committee for Dietary Supplements.

Introduction

Analytical method development will be a critical component of dietary supplement manufacturing in coming years, as good manufacturing practices (GMPs) are implemented. This *Handbook of Analytical Methods for Dietary Supplements* is a convenient reference source that provides a starting point for laboratories to develop and validate analytical testing methods for dietary supplements. This handbook is not meant to be a comprehensive tome on every analytical method published for every dietary supplement or botanical raw material. Rather, it offers a sampling of methods along with appropriate validation data, if known, about the most common supplements in the marketplace.

Dietary supplements are everywhere today. From multivitamins, to nutraceuticals, "natural" weight-loss aids, and herbal energy boosters, dietary supplements can be found on the Internet and in grocery stores, pharmacies, convenience marts, and specialty shops. Traditionally, the government has minimally enforced regulations for dietary supplements, and it was not until 2003 that the Food and Drug Administration (FDA) proposed GMPs to define methods, equipment, facilities, and controls for ensuring quality. Testing of dietary supplements for active ingredients or marker compounds has often taken a haphazard, shotgun approach, and few official, validated methods are available. The enormous variety of formulations on the market means that even the few official test methods published by the United States Pharmacopeial Convention or AOAC International do not work for some products.

GMPs Intend to Ensure Products Are Tested

FDA's Proposed Rule on Dietary Supplement GMPs, issued on March 13, 2003, was a long time coming—and after you read it all, it's clear why. In October 1994, Congress passed the Dietary Supplement Health and Education Act (DSHEA), an amendment to the Federal Food, Drug and Cosmetic Act (FFDCA) designed to regulate dietary supplements. Among other provisions, it authorized FDA to establish GMPs for dietary supplements modeled after those for foods. In November 1995, the dietary supplement industry delivered to FDA a document detailing state-of-the-art practices in manufacturing dietary supplements, which FDA published in February 1997 in an Advanced Notice of Proposed Rule Making (ANPRM), along with a series of questions FDA wanted the industry to answer before moving further. Thus began the rulemaking process. After six years of prompting and prodding from the industry, FDA finally performed the next step by issuing the Proposed Rule in 2003.

To look at the matter from FDA's perspective, you must understand what these GMPs intend to accomplish. They guarantee neither the safety nor efficacy of these products. GMPs do assure, however, that the products are tested to ensure that they meet label claims and that manufacturers can prove they have been tested. Think that sounds odd? Generally, the FDA is concerned with safety and efficacy, but all that is required here is verification of identity and purity. FDA's opening comments in the Proposed Rule state the following:

"The provisions would require manufacturers to evaluate the identity, purity, quality, strength, and composition of their dietary ingredients and dietary supplements." [68 FR, No. 49, page 12158.]

With the forthcoming GMPs proposed by the FDA, the need for analytical testing of dietary supplements is coming to the forefront. Manufacturers will need to verify the quality of their incoming raw materials and ensure that their finished products meet label claims. Contract testing laboratories will be challenged to develop and validate methods for the wide range of supplements that will be coming through their doors.

As for the required amount of testing, the Proposed Rule contains only one specific mandate: you must test the final dietary ingredient or dietary supplement product. FDA does, however, recommend that you test incoming materials before sending them through to manufacture the finished product—which makes good business sense. Further, FDA wants you to perform testing on your packaging materials to confirm their suitability for direct product contact (e.g., bottles, blister packs, etc.). This requirement, implied in the Proposed Rule, comes about because FDA says you cannot accept a supplier's Certificate of Analysis, which describes quality control data for a particular batch of product, as proof of such conformance. If the finished product cannot be tested once all the ingredients are blended in the final form, you are required to test the incoming materials and the product during the manufacturing process.

Challenges in Testing

Because FDA's proposed GMPs attempt to minimize the testing you must perform to ensure that products deliver the strength, composition, and purity indicated on the label, the quality of analysis is key. Based on what is written in the preamble to the Proposed Rule, key points from which are summarized below, FDA perceives this to be a relatively simple task.

FDA is unaware of any instances where tests do not exist for dietary supplements. (However, FDA is not specific about what kind of tests.)

FDA allows the use of unofficial, validated methods (i.e., methods not from FDA or AOAC International, a scientific association committed to valid analytical results.) You do not need to perform the testing yourself; you can have an outside laboratory do it for you.

The only challenge you may face is difficulty in testing your finished product matrix.

However, FDA's unawareness of a lack of methods is probably because it has not asked the dietary supplements industry whether such tests exist—nor has the industry volunteered the information. The truth is, appropriate methods are not available for testing all dietary supplements. FDA is beginning to address this issue by contracting with AOAC International to develop and validate methods for various dietary supplements, but the scope of the contract addresses only a dozen or so of the most popular supplement ingredients. Furthermore, the timeframe of the contract (5 years) means that official methods for analyzing some of these ingredients will not be available for several years.

This *Handbook,* in addition to putting forth a sampling of analytical testing methods, offers guidelines and insights on developing dietary supplements methods, such as stability and solubility issues, detection methods, and possible interferences or adulterants. For many ingredients, no published papers exist regarding their testing in dietary supplements. In these cases, we provide chromatographic methods used for testing in biological or botanical matrices, along with possible approaches for testing in dietary supplements.

Method Validation for Dietary Supplements

The goal of any analytical method, whether for measuring pesticides in food, an active ingredient in a pharmaceutical product, or a marker compound in a botanical raw material, is to provide accurate, reproducible results. And how do you know that a method yields accurate, reproducible results: by being validated—that is, shown to be valid for its intended purpose.

But what exactly is validation, and how do you go about proving that a method is valid for its intended purpose? This topic has become of central importance in the dietary supplement industry as manufacturers are called on to support their ingredient label claims—a process that requires analytical testing, both of raw materials and finished products.

In the dietary supplement industry, however, it is not unusual for two different laboratories to test the same material for the same compound and obtain two completely different results. Often the difference in results can be attributed to:

- Differences in sample extraction procedures
- Purity of reference standards
- Selectivity of method
- Scope and applicability of the method

Three out of these four areas are addressed directly during the method validation process. Knowing the purity of reference standards is not specifically a validation issue, but it is critical in obtaining accurate and reproducible results.

An entire book could be devoted to method validation for dietary supplements. In this section, it is not the goal to provide exhaustive instructions for validating a method, but rather to give guidelines for analysts to follow and to point out issues to consider when performing or assessing a method validation. No magic formulas or easy recipes exist for validating analytical test methods for dietary supplements—every method is unique and presents its own unique challenges. The person overseeing the validation is responsible for developing strategies to ensure that the results obtained are reliable.

Performance Characteristics

When a method is validated, certain qualities about the method are measured; these are referred to as performance characteristics. Performance characteristics are "the functional qualities and statistical measures of the degree of reliability exhibited by the method under specified operating conditions."[1] They answer the question, "How good is the method?" Performance characteristics are defined by functional qualities and performance limits. Functional qualities include:

- Scope and applicability
- Selectivity
- Precision (measured as the variability)
- Reliability (measured as the recovery)
- Range

Performance limits are the limits or ranges within which each functional quality measurement must fall for the method to be considered valid. For each analytical method, the analyst must come up with a series of experiments to determine the corresponding functional qualities.

It is important to realize that there are different levels of method validation. The most basic level of validation is within a single laboratory. Results from single-laboratory validation apply to a specific operator (or operators) in a specific laboratory using specific equipment. These results provide no information about how a method will perform once it goes outside the validating laboratory.

Many of the monographs in this *Handbook*, by necessity, are based on single-laboratory validation data. The reader must be cautious in assuming that these results can be repeated by other laboratories. Differences in the level of training of personnel, familiarity with the method, differences in equipment manufacturer and design, and individual laboratory techniques can lead to differences in method performance between laboratories.

Validating a method within a single laboratory is very useful if the method will not be used outside that laboratory, which may occur when proprietary products are being tested, a very limited number of samples is to be tested, the method is being used for research and development purposes, or the method is being used for quality control of a single item by a single producer.

Performing a single-laboratory validation on a method is also the first step in going up to the next level, an interlaboratory validation. If the laboratory that developed and attempted to validate the method in-house cannot get the method to meet the required performance limits, the chances of outside laboratories obtaining accurate and reproducible results with that method are slim. If the single-laboratory validation results for a method look good, it bodes well for the success of that method when that method is used in another laboratory.

Interlaboratory validation is a process showing that at least two different laboratories can obtain reproducible results on the same sample set using the same method. At least two, and sometimes more, laboratories are involved in an interlaboratory validation, a process that often occurs between a raw material supplier and a manufacturer, for example, or between a manufacturer and a third-party contract analytical laboratory.

The gold standard of method validation is the collaborative study. A collaborative study requires at least eight participating laboratories and often involves more. Procedures in the *Official Methods of Analysis* published by the AOAC International have undergone full collaborative studies. In a collaborative study, samples are sent out as blind duplicates to participating laboratories, which are not given the identities or expected concentrations of analyte in the samples. A method that has survived the collaborative study can be expected to do well in most competent laboratories.

Scope and Applicability

The first step in validating any method, and possibly the most overlooked step, is to define the scope and applicability of a method. This involves answering the following questions:

- What is (are) the analyte(s)?
- What is (are) the matrix (or matrices)?
- What are the expected concentration ranges of the analyte(s) in the matrices?

For pharmaceutical products, it is usually a straightforward process. The method will be used to test active ingredient X in matrix Y. Because there will usually be only one form of the active ingredient in one matrix (perhaps at several different strengths), it is easy to define the scope and applicability of the method.

For dietary supplements, particularly those that contain botanical products, it is another story. When someone says, "I need a method for Ginkgo biloba," what are they really asking for? Ginkgo biloba, for example, contains numerous marker compounds: hypericin, bilobalide, and ginkgolide A, ginkgolide B, ginkgolide C, ginkgolide J, as well as flavonoids such as quercetin, isorhamnetin and kaempferol. Contract manufacturers and contract analytical laboratories might find Ginkgo biloba products in tablets, capsules, softgels, and tinctures, alone or in combination with other botanical products, vitamins, or minerals. Such variations are typical of many botanicals found in dietary supplements.

Key Challenges

The scope and applicability of a method will necessarily be determined by the intended end use of the method. Will the method be used to support label claims, to meet regulatory requirements, to address safety and efficacy issues, or to support a marketing strategy?

As if this is not confusing enough, the analytes must be defined. You can develop methods to target specific ginsenosides in ginseng, for example, or you can develop a method to quantify total ginsenosides. A popular method for testing St. John's wort for hypericin is a spectrophotometric method, which quantifies total dianthrones, not just hypericin, and yields very different results from those of a high-performance liquid chromatography (HPLC) method that targets hypericin specifically. Many marker compounds exist as glycosides in the botanical. Ginkgo biloba contains more than 20 glycosides of the flavonoids quercetin, kaempferol, and isorhamnetin, yet on hydrolysis, only these three components are left, which are very easily quantified. Is a method needed that tests for each of the individual glycosides, or just the aglycones?

For many products in this book, the literature contains no methods for their analysis in dietary supplements and therefore this *Handbook* includes methods developed for biological samples (plasma, urine, tissue, etc.) or environmental samples. Although these often provide a good starting place for developing methods for dietary supplements, major modifications likely will be required. If laboratories test a dietary supplement product using a method designed for biological samples, you should be very suspicious of the results, unless the laboratory supplies sufficient validation data for your matrix type.

The Proper Breadth

When defining the scope and applicability of a method, do not make them broader than necessary. While it is nice to have a method that works for "everything," a universal method can often be complex and cumbersome, and the work required to validate such a method becomes prohibitive. Focus on the sample matrices and specific analytes that you will be dealing with immediately. You can always add analytes and matrices down the road if needed. At the same time, do not make the scope and applicability so narrow that the method cannot handle the samples for which it was designed.

Selectivity

Selectivity is the term used to describe a method's ability to accurately quantify an analyte in the presence of matrix components. These components include other active ingredients, excipients, degradation products, or compounds that could possibly be used as adulterants.

The selectivity of a method can be achieved through several means: chromatographic separation, selective extraction of analyte(s) from sample matrix, enzymatic or chemical reactions, and/or selective detection techniques. Often a combination of these techniques is used to obtain the necessary selectivity.

For example, a method might use solid-phase extraction to remove one or more classes of compounds from the sample matrix, followed by liquid chromatography to separate the analyte from other remaining components, with detection and quantitation by fluorometry. Interfering components can cause systematic errors (bias) in the results.

Matrix Blank

The selectivity of a method can be demonstrated in several ways. The chosen approach often depends on the analyte and sample matrix. Injecting a "matrix blank" into the HPLC system and showing there are no interfering peaks is one technique. The matrix blank is usually a representative sample that does not contain detectable levels of the analyte and undergoes the identical sample preparation procedure as an actual sample. In pharmaceutical analysis, this would be like injecting a placebo preparation.

For botanical raw materials, however, true matrix blanks do not exist. How do you obtain a true ginseng extract that does not contain ginsenosides? In some cases, you may be able to substitute a closely related species that does not contain the marker compound of interest. For example, *Ephedra nevadensis*, a species of ephedra that does not contain ephedrine alkaloids, could be used as a matrix blank for a method used to determine ephedrine alkaloids in *Ephedra sinica*. Often, however, it is impossible to find a surrogate species to serve as a matrix blank, and other techniques must be used to demonstrate selectivity.

For finished products, one approach to show selectivity is to find the most complex dietary supplement on the market that does not contain the ingredient of interest, and use that as a matrix blank. Multivitamins that contain botanical extracts often work well for that purpose.

Peak Purity

Photodiode-array (PDA) detection and/or mass spectroscopic (MS) detection are useful for determining peak purity by showing there are no "hidden" peaks under the analyte peak. Be cautious about relying solely on PDA detection to determine peak purity, however, because closely related compounds that may coelute often have identical UV spectra. Using PDA and MS detection in tandem is often sufficient to prove selectivity of a method. The selectivity should be demonstrated on each sample matrix specified in the scope and applicability of the method.

If PDA or MS detection is not available and you can spend the extra time, another approach to demonstrating peak purity is to collect the fractions containing the analyte peaks as they elute from the detector. An orthogonal analytical technique, such as thin-layer chromatography (TLC) or electrophoresis, can then be used to analyze the collected peaks to show that no other compounds have coeluted.

Precision

Precision is a measure of the repeatability of a method and is usually expressed as a standard deviation (or more commonly, a relative standard deviation) of replicate analyses. It is an expression of the random error associated with a method.

Different ways to measure the repeatability of a method include the repeatability between:

- Replicate injections of the same sample solution (instrument precision).
- Replicate preparations of the same sample prepared on the same day (within-day precision).
- Replicate preparations of the same sample prepared on separate days (between-day precision).
- Replicate preparations of the same sample prepared by different analysts (between-analyst precision).

Measuring Repeatability

Once a method is used in a second laboratory, interlaboratory precision can be measured. In a collaborative study, in which a statistically meaningful number of laboratories participate, the reproducibility of the method can be measured. The terms "repeatability" and "reproducibility" are often used interchangeably, but they are in fact different measurements. Reproducibility refers to results obtained when different laboratories analyze the same samples under a variety of normal test conditions: different analysts, different days, and different instruments.

Repeatability, which refers to measurement within one laboratory, gives the laboratory a good indication of how well results of multiple tests on the same sample generated within that laboratory will agree with each other. A laboratory can then assign a "confidence interval" to a reported value, such as "10.0 mg ± 0.2 mg." Unfortunately, many laboratories' certificates of analysis do not include this information, and customers therefore have no idea what the range of the actual result might be.

The key to determining meaningful repeatability measurements is to perform enough experiments on a sample. For pharmaceuticals, the United States Pharmacopeia guidelines for validation of compendial methods recommend at least five replicate sample preparations on at least two days. Following this guideline, however, yields very limited data on between-day precision.

AOAC International guidelines recommend that when the number of replicate sample preparations within-day is multiplied by the number of days, the total number should not be less than 10. Not only will five replicate sample preparations on two days fulfill this requirement, but two replicate sample preparations on five different days will also do the same. Conducting precision studies over five days can be impractical for a laboratory, however, so a happy medium is often used; four or five replicate sample preparations over three or four days usually works well. The more data generated, the better. One cannot do too many experiments, only too few. It is also important to perform the repeatability experiments on each sample type covered by the scope of the method.

Acceptable Results

Once a laboratory has conducted sufficient precision studies, the results must be interpreted. Three useful pieces of information can be culled from all the precision data: within-day precision of the method, between-day precision of the method, and total precision of the method. Then analysis of variance (ANOVA) calculations can be performed on the data, which is easily done using one of the many available software packages, including Microsoft Excel.

What is considered acceptable precision? That is, what performance limits should be set? The limits depend on the concentration of analyte in the sample matrix. The lower the concentration of the analyte in the sample matrix, the larger the variances. Relative standard deviations (RSDs) for reproducibility studies (RSD_R) can be predicted using the Horwitz equation[2]:

$$\text{Predicted } RSD_R = 2C^{-0.15}$$

where C is the concentration of the analyte in the sample matrix, expressed as a mass fraction (Horwitz). From this equation, and the actual reproducibility data obtained in a collaborative study, a HORRAT (Horwitz ratio) value can be calculated:

$$\text{HORRAT} = \text{Actual } RSD_R \;/\; \text{Predicted } RSD_R$$

Approximate predicted RSD_R values for varying analyte concentrations in the sample matrix are:

Concentration	Predicted RSD_R
100%	1.0%
10%	1.4%
1%	2.0%
0.1%	2.8%
0.01%	4.0%
0.001%	5.6%
0.0001% (1 ppm)	8.0%

Typical acceptable HORRAT values are between 0.5 and 2. Values greater than 2 indicate that there may be a problem with the method: incomplete extraction of the sample, degradation of the analyte, the presence of matrix interferences, or other method gremlins that are not easily identified.

This Horwitz equation calculates predicted RSDs for reproducibility studies, that is, precision measurements obtained with a large number of collaborative laboratories. Often one does not have the luxury of performing a collaborative study on a method and must rely on single-laboratory validation data. What types of RSDs can be expected for a single-laboratory repeatability study? Predicted RSDs for within-lab precision studies (RSD_R) are one-half the value calculated for reproducibility RSDs (Horwitz). Acceptable HORRAT values are two-thirds those calculated for reproducibility studies, or between 0.3 and 1.3.

Accuracy

The ultimate goal of any analytical method is to produce results that are close to the true value—a concept referred to as "accuracy." The difference between the result as determined using the method and the true value is the "bias" of the method. How do you know what the true value is? For most pharmaceutical products, performing a spike recovery experiment is sufficient: a placebo matrix is spiked with a known amount of the active ingredient and the spiked placebo is assayed using the method. The accuracy of the method is then expressed as percent recovery. This approach also works for simple, nonbotanical dietary supplements, like some vitamins, or simple chemical ingredients, like melatonin and glucosamine.

Spike Recovery of Botanicals

For products containing botanical materials, however, the situation is much more complex. Obtaining a "placebo" of a botanical is often impossible, and spiking a compound onto a negative control does not always imitate the environment that the marker compound experiences in a real sample, particularly if the botanical product is a ground herb with cellular material still intact. Although spike recovery studies can provide some useful information about the accuracy of the method in situations like this, other techniques should also be used to help verify the accuracy.

In botanical materials, spike recovery studies involve spiking an appropriate negative control (placebo) with known amounts of analyte at different levels, covering the expected concentration range in typical samples. The analytes are usually spiked at levels of about 200% of the target concentration, at the target concentration, and at a lower level, such as the limit of quantitation (LOQ) of the method, or whatever the lowest significant level is expected to be.

At least seven replicates at each spike level should be performed over several days, so that within-day and between-day precision of recovery levels can be calculated. This will help isolate the random error, measured by the precision, from the systematic error, measured by the bias. A common approach is to spike at three different levels in triplicate on three separate days. If a negative control is not available, the method of standard addition can be used to help determine accuracy; however, the level of analyte in this case will always be higher than the target value.

Using Certified Reference Materials

Certified reference materials (CRMs) containing known quantities of the marker compounds of interest can be used to determine the accuracy of a method. The CRM is tested using the proposed method, and the bias of the method is determined by comparing the actual result with the stated concentration. These reference materials are distributed by national metrological laboratories, such as the National Institute of Standards and Technology (NIST), or by commercial suppliers. A certified reference material will be highly characterized, and the marker compound concentration will be known to a high degree of accuracy. Unfortunately, the number of standard reference materials available for botanical products is limited, so material needed for a particular method may not be available.

Acceptable recoveries depend on the concentration of analyte in the matrix. They are summarized in the following table (AOAC International):

Concentration	Recovery Limits
100%	98% to 101%
10%	95% to 102%
1%	92% to 105%
0.1%	90% to 108%
0.01%	85% to 110%
0.001% (10 ppm)	80% to 115%
0.0001% (1 ppm)	75% to 120%
0.000001% (10 ppb)	70% to 125%

Recoveries above the upper limit indicate possible matrix interferences. Recoveries below the lower limit indicate incomplete extraction, poor analyte solubility, or analyte decomposition. One way to determine the extraction efficiency and analyte solubility is to quantitatively remove half of the sample solution from the flask in which the stock sample solution is contained, and add that same volume of extraction solvent back into the flask. The analyte concentration should be exactly half the original concentration. If the analyte is found to be more than half the original concentration, then the sample was either incompletely extracted the first time or the analyte has limited solubility in the extraction solvent and the procedure may need to be modified.

Range

The range is a function of the accuracy and precision of the method together with the scope and applicability. Range refers to the concentration range of analyte in the sample matrix that can be quantified accurately and reproducibly. Determining the range of a method may not be important if the analyte concentration is expected to be within a very narrow concentration range, but determining the range of a method is critical for dietary supplements containing botanical products and for methods designed to test a wide variety of supplements. It is not uncommon for laboratories to report analyte values at levels well below those demonstrated by the method validation. These results should be viewed as highly questionable until experiments have shown the results to be valid at those levels.

Range is usually demonstrated through accuracy and precision experiments. The range of the method should be defined at the same time as the scope and applicability, while spiked recovery and repeatability studies should be performed at or near the extremes of these ranges.

Conclusions

This brief overview of method validation for dietary supplements touched on issues and problems involved with validating methods in the dietary supplement industry. Contract analytical laboratories dealing with an enormous variety of formulations (and thus sample matrices) with a wide range of analyte concentrations face a big challenge. Because validating methods for each formulation becomes impractical, creative approaches are sometimes needed to show that a method is valid.

References

1. AOAC International Guidelines for Single Laboratory Validation of Chemical Methods for Dietary Supplements and Botanicals, April 2003.
2. Horwitz W. Evaluation of analytical methods used for regulation of foods and drugs. *Anal Chem.* 1982;54:67–76.

Key Terms

Accuracy: Producing results that are close to the true value.

Collaborative study: The gold standard of method validation, in which eight or more laboratories analyze samples they receive as blind duplicates; they are not given the identities or expected concentrations of analyte in the samples.

Functional qualities: Aspects that define performance characteristics, including scope and applicability, selectivity, precision (measured as the variability), reliability (measured as the recovery), and range. For each analytical method, the analyst must come up with a series of experiments to determine the functional qualities.

Interlaboratory validation: A process showing that at least two different laboratories obtained reproducible results on the same sample set using the same method.

Matrix blank: A representative sample that does not contain detectable levels of the analyte and that is treated to the identical sample preparation procedure as an actual sample.

Performance characteristics: Functional qualities and statistical measures of the degree of reliability exhibited by the method under specified operating conditions. These characteristics answer the question, "How good is the method?"

Performance limits: The limits or ranges within which each functional quality measurement must fall for the method to be considered valid.

Precision: A measure of the repeatability of a method, usually expressed as a standard deviation (or more commonly, a relative standard deviation) of replicate analyses.

Range: The concentration range of analyte in the sample matrix that can accurately and reproducibly be quantified. Range is a function of the accuracy and precision of the method as well as the scope and applicability.

Selectivity: The term used to describe a method's ability to accurately quantify an analyte in the presence of matrix components.

Spike recovery: An experiment in which a placebo matrix is spiked with a known amount of the active ingredient. The spiked placebo is then assayed using the analytical method. The accuracy of the method is expressed as percent recovery.

Monographs

ARTICHOKE

Description

Botanical name: *Cynara scolymus* L.

Common names: Cynara, globe artichoke

Parts of plant used: Dried leaves

Uses: As a choleretic.

Mode of Action

Long known as an herbal medicine, the dried leaves of artichoke have been used for their choleretic properties since remote times.[1] In various pharmacological test systems, artichoke leaf extracts have shown antibacterial, antioxidative, anti-HIV, bile-expelling, and hepatoprotective properties; urinative activity; and inhibition of cholesterol biosynthesis and LDL oxidation.[2–10] The mono- and dicaffeoylquinic acid derivatives and flavonoids are believed to be bioactive compounds in artichoke, although there are no supporting data.

Chemical Markers

Artichoke leaves have been studied extensively and found to be a rich source of polyphenolic compounds, with mono- and dicaffeoylquinic acids and flavonoids as the major chemical components.[11] The main caffeoylquinic acid derivatives in artichoke leaves are chlorogenic acid and 1,5-dicaffeoylquinic acid, which can be converted to 1,3-dicaffeoylquinic acid during extraction and processing. Other compounds identified in artichoke include sesquiterpenoid lactones and flavonoids (e.g., luteolin-7-O-glucoside, luteolin-7-O-rutinoside). The caffeoylquinic derivatives are used as marker compounds for quality control of artichoke leaf extracts.

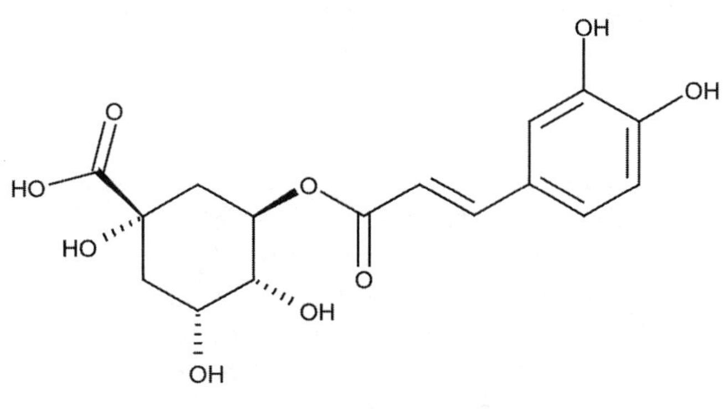

Chlorogenic acid

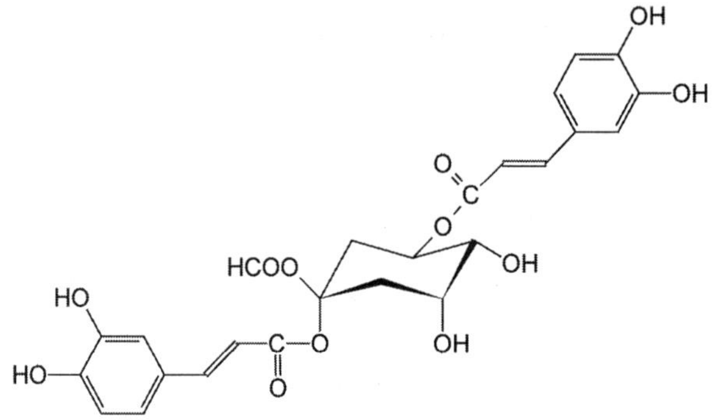

1,5-Dicaffeoylquinic acid (cynarin)

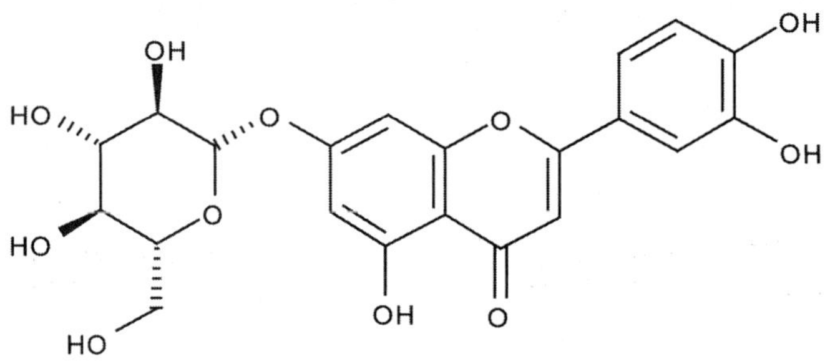

Cynaroside (luteolin-7-O-glucoside)

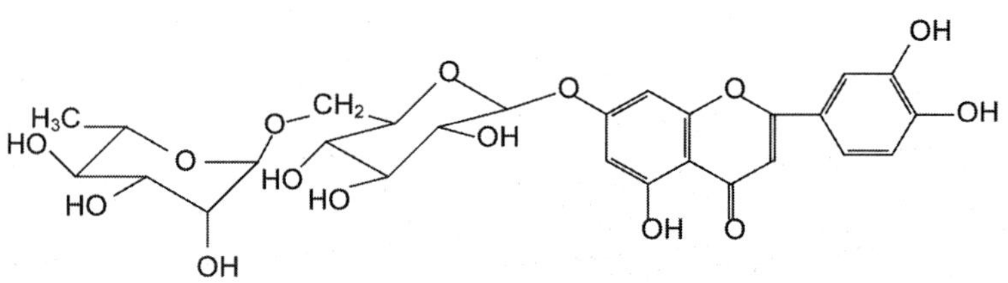

Luteolin-7-O-rutinoside

Major phenolic compounds identified in artichoke leaves.

Methods of Analysis

Various methods have been used to analyze the phenolic compounds in artichoke, including colorimetry, reversed-phase HPLC (RP-HPLC), micellar electrokinetic capillary chromatography, and TLC.[12–18] HPLC is the most accepted analytical method for caffeoylquinic acid derivatives.

The extraction solvent is key in the analysis of caffeoylquinic acid derivatives. Various solvents have been tried for extracting compounds from artichoke leaves, with 60% methanol found to be best.[11]

Method 1: The method of Bilia et al.[19] can be used to analyze chlorogenic acid, cynarin 1,5-dicaffeoylquinic acid, isochlorogenic acid, luteolin-7-O-glucoside (cynaroside), and luteolin-7-O-rutinoside.

Sample preparation: Prepare samples in 60% and 40% methanol.

Chromatography

Column: LiChrosorb RP-18, 5-μm, 250 × 4.0 mm with LiChrosorb RP-18 guard column, 5 μm, 10 × 4 mm.

Mobile phase: Solvent A = water (adjusted to pH 3 with phosphoric acid), solvent B = acetonitrile.

Gradient:

Time (minutes)	%A	%B
0	88	12
10	82	18
15	82	18
30	55	45
35	0	100
42	0	100
50	88	12

Flow rate: 1.3 mL/minute

Injection volume: 25 μL

Detection wavelength: 350 nm

Column temperature: 26°C

Validation data:

Linearity: 0.10 to 2.5 mcg with a correlation coefficient greater than 0.99.

Accuracy: Not specified

Precision: Each of the seven compounds had an RSD that was less than 3.7%.

Selectivity: Peak identification was determined against standards.

Ruggedness: Not specified

Robustness: Not specified

LOD/LOQ: Not specified

Method 2: The method of Wang et al.[11] was used to analyze cynarin, 1-caffeoylquinic acid, chlorogenic acid, luteolin-7-O-glucoside, and luteolin-7-O-rutinoside in artichoke leaves and to analyze two additional compounds, narirutin (naringenin-7-O-rutinoside) and apigenin-7-rutinoside (isorhoifolin), in artichoke heads (flowers).

Sample preparation: Extract 500 mg of dried leaves with 70 mL of 60% methanol by sonicating for 25 minutes. Cool the sample to room temperature and dilute to 100 mL with 60% methanol.

Chromatography

Column: Phenomenex Prodigy ODS3, 5 µm, 150 × 3.2 mm.
Mobile phase: Solvent A = water (with 0.2% phosphoric acid), solvent B = acetonitrile.
Gradient: 6%B linear to 30%B in 20 minutes, hold at 30%B for an additional 5 minutes.
Flow rate: 1.2 mL/minute
Injection volume: 10 µL
Detection wavelength: 330 nm

Validation data:

Linearity: 1.08 to 216 mcg/mL for chlorogenic acid, 1.1 to 220 mcg/mL for 1-caffeoylquinic acid, 0.92 to 184 mcg/mL for luteolin-7-O-rutinoside, 1.06 to 212 mcg/mL for luteolin-7-O-glucoside, and 1.24 to 248 mcg/mL for cynarin; the correlation coefficient for each compound was 1.
Accuracy: The percentage recoveries were from 97.6 to 100.7 for these five compounds.
Precision: Each compound had an RSD that was less than 2.33%.
Selectivity: Peak identification was determined against standards.
Ruggedness: Not specified
Robustness: Not specified
LOD/LOQ: Not specified

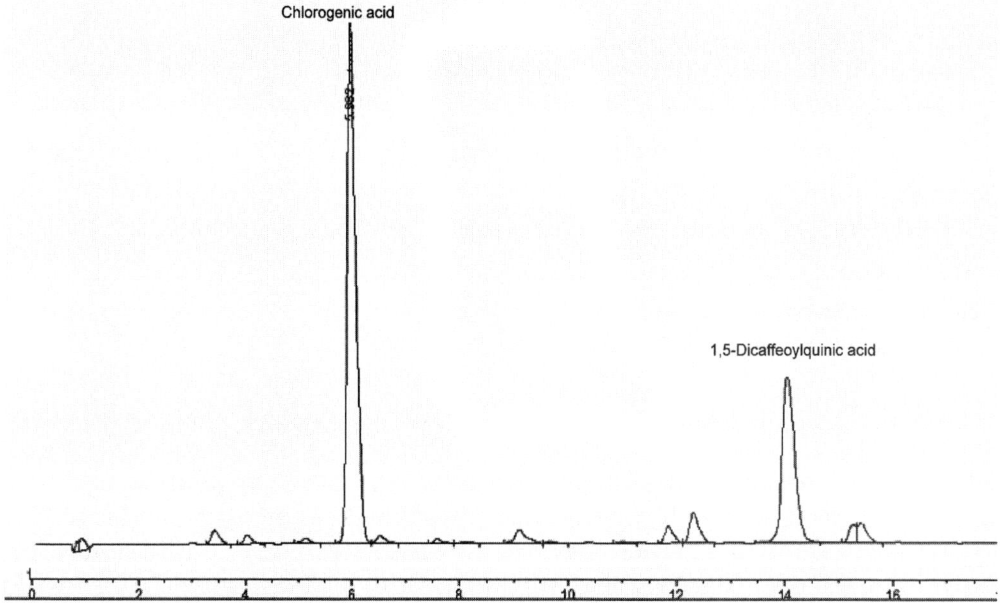

Representative HPLC chromatogram of artichoke run by method 2.

References

1. Bruneton J. *Pharmacognosy, Phytochemistry, Medicinal Plants.* Secaucus, NJ: Lavoisier Publishing; 1995:218–9.
2. Alamanni MC, Cossu M. Antioxidant activity of the extracts of the edible part of artichoke (*Cynara scolymus* L.) var spinoso sardo. *Ital J Food Sci.* 2003;15:187–95.
3. Dranik LI, Dolganenko LG, Slapke J, et al. Chemical composition and medical usage of *Cynara scolymus* L. *Rastit Resur.* 1996;32:98–104.
4. Martino V, Caffini N, Phillipson JD, et al. Identification and characterization of antimicrobial components in leaf extracts of globe artichoke (*Cynara scolymus* L.). *Acta Horticulturae.* 1999;501:111–4.
5. McDougall B, King PJ, Wu BW, et al. Dicaffeoylquinic acid and dicaffeoyltartaric acid are selective inhibitors of human immunodeficiency virus type 1 integrase. *Antimicrob Agents Chemother.* 1998;42:140–6.
6. Kraft K. Artichoke leaf extract—recent findings reflecting effects on lipid metabolism, liver and gastrointestinal tracts. *Phytomedicine.* 1997;4:369–78.
7. Brown JE, Rice-Evans CA. Luteolin-rich artichoke extract protects low density lipoprotein from oxidation *in vitro. Free Radic Res.* 1998;29:247–55.
8. Gebhardt R. Prevention of taurolithocholate-induced hepatic bile canalicular distortions by HPLC-characterized extracts of artichoke (*Cynara scolymus* L.) leaves. *Planta Med.* 2002; 68:776–9.
9. Gebhardt R. Antioxidative and protective properties of extracts from leaves of artichoke (*Cynara scolymus* L.) against hydroperoxide-induced oxidative stress in cultured rat hepatocytes. *Toxicol Appl Pharmacol.* 1997;144:279–86.
10. Perez-Garcia F, Adzet T, Canigueral S. Activity of artichoke leaf extract on reactive oxygen species in human leukocytes. *Free Radic Res.* 2000;33:661–5.
11. Wang M, Simon JE, Aviles IF, et al. Analysis of antioxidative phenolic compounds in artichoke (*Cynara scolymus* L.). *J Agric Food Chem.* 2003;51:601–8.
12. Sevcikova P, Glatz Z, Slanina J. Analysis of artichoke (*Cynara cardunculus* L.) extract by means of micellar electrokinetic capillary chromatography. *Electrophoresis.* 2002;23: 249–52.
13. Krawczyk A. Standardization of raw material and extract of artichoke (*Cynara scolymus* L.). *Herba Pol.* 2001;47:130–6.
14. Hammouda FM, Self El-Nasr MM, Ismail SI, et al. Quantitative determination of the active constituents in Egyptian cultivated *Cynara scolymus* L. *Int J Pharmacogn.* 1993;31: 299–304.
15. Debenedetti SL, Palacios PS, Wilson EG, et al. HPLC analysis of caffeoylquinic acids content in Argentine medicinal plants. *Acta Horticulturae.* 1993;333:191–9.
16. Slanina J, Taborska E, Musil P. Determination of cynarine in the decoctions of the artichoke (*Cynara cardunculus* L.) by the HPLC method. *Cesko-Slov Farm.* 1993;42:265–8.
17. Ben-Hod G, Basnizki Y, Zohary D, et al. Cynarin and chlorogenic acid content in germinating seeds of globe artichoke (*Cynara scolymus* L.). *J Genet Breed.* 1992;46:63–9.
18. Adzet T, Puigmacia M. High-performance liquid chromatography of caffeoylquinic acid derivatives of *Cynara scolymus* L. leaves. *J Chromatogr.* 1985;348:447–52.
19. Bilia AR, Bergonzi MC, Mazzi G, et al. Analysis and stability of the constituents of artichoke and St. John's wort tinctures by HPLC–DAD and HPLC–MS. *Drug Dev Ind Pharm.* 2002;28:609–19.

ASCORBIC ACID

Description

Chemical names: 3-Oxo-L-gulofuranolactone; L-3-ketothreohexuronic acid; 2-oxo-L-threo-hexono-1,4-lactone-2,3-enediol

Common names: L-Ascorbic acid, vitamin C

Molecular weight: 176.13

Chemical formula: $C_6H_8O_6$

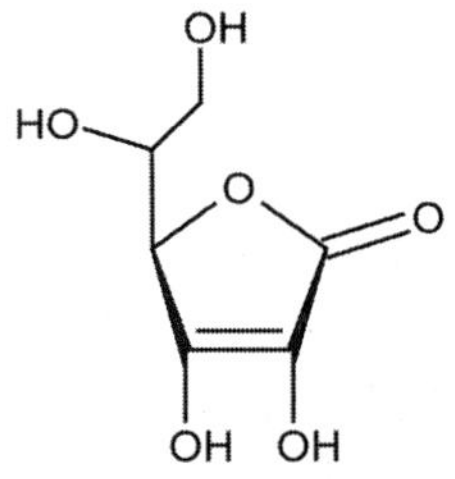

Ascorbic acid

Solubility: Highly water soluble, moderately soluble in alcohol and glycerol. Insoluble in ether, chloroform, benzene, and other nonpolar organic solvents.

Other physical/chemical data:

$pKa_1 = 4.17$, $pKa_2 = 11.57$

UV max = 245 nm (acidic solution, ε = 12,200), 265 nm (neutral solution, ε = 16,600)

$[\alpha]_D = +20.5°$ to $+21.5°$ at 25°C (c = 1)

Melting point = 190°C to 192°C (decomposition)

Uses: Prevention and treatment of vitamin C deficiency; as an antimicrobial and antioxidant in food products.

Mode of Action

Ascorbic acid is an effective reducing agent. It helps maintain the activity of the enzyme prolyl hydroxylase, which is necessary for the synthesis of collagen, by keeping the iron atom at its active site in the ferrous state. Ascorbic acid also acts as a free-radical scavenger within cells.

Methods of Analysis

Many methods have been published for the analysis of ascorbic acid in dietary supplements and foods. These methods include reversed-phase and ion-exchange chromatography, spectrophotometry, titrimetry, and fluorometry.

Method 1: Most analytical methods for ascorbic acid focus on food, beverages, tissue, and plasma rather than dietary supplements. Nevertheless, these methods can often be adapted easily to the analysis of dietary supplements.

Sample and standard preparation: Because of its high solubility in water, ascorbic acid is usually extracted with or dissolved in an aqueous medium. Unfortunately, ascorbic acid is readily oxidized in aqueous solution to dehydroascorbic acid, and it can also be hydrolyzed to 2,3-diketo-L-gulonic acid. Dehydroascorbic acid can be converted back to ascorbic acid by reducing agents; however, the degradation of ascorbic acid to 2,3-diketo-L-gulonic acid is not reversible. The presence of metals in solution increases the rate of oxidative degradation,[1] and heat, light, and basic pH also increase the degradation rate. Therefore, any sample and standard preparation technique should be developed with the goal of minimizing degradation. Low actinic glassware should be used, and the solution pH should be kept acidic. Often metaphosphoric acid is added to the diluent to maintain an acidic pH; it also slows down metal-catalyzed oxidation. Reducing agents and edetic acid (EDTA) can be added to solutions of ascorbic acid to minimize degradation during analysis. Dithiothreitol,[2] homocysteine,[3] L-cysteine,[4] and tris[2-carboxyethyl]phosphine[5] have all been used as reductants to prevent oxidation of ascorbic acid.

Chromatography: Lykkesfeldt[5] used reversed-phase HPLC with ion-pairing and electrochemical detection to assay ascorbic acid in biological samples. Tris[2-carboxyethyl]phosphine (0.25 mM) was used as a reducing agent in the standard and sample solutions.

Column: Phenomenex Luna C18, 3 μm, 150 × 4.6 mm, equipped with SecurityGuard C18 column.

Mobile phase: Solvent A = 100 mM NaH_2PO_4, 100 mM sodium acetate monohydrate, 1.0 mM EDTA, and 0.189 mM *n*-dodecyltrimethylammonium chloride in water; solvent B = 36.6 μM tetraoctylammonium bromide; pH was adjusted to 5.4 with phosphoric acid; 75%A/25%B was used.

Flow rate: 0.6 mL/minute

Column temperature: 30°C

Injection volume: 10 μL

Detection: Coulometric, dual cell (–200 mV and +300 mV)

Validation data:

Linearity: 5 to 100 μM ascorbic acid, $r^2>0.99$.

Accuracy: 102.1% recovery of spiked plasma compared to linearity standards.

Precision: <1% RSD (six spiked samples)

Selectivity: Peak identification was achieved by quantitative oxidation of ascorbic acid with ascorbic acid oxidase.

Ruggedness: Between-days coefficient of variation less than 3.5%.

Robustness: Not determined

LOD/LOQ: Not determined

References

1. Tannenbaum SR, Young VR. Vitamins and minerals. In: Fennema OR, ed. *Food Chemistry.* New York: Marcel Dekker; 1985:477.
2. Doner LW, Hicks KB. High-performance liquid chromatographic separation of ascorbic acid, erythorbic acid, dehydroascorbic acid, dehydroerythorbic acid, diketogulonic acid, and diketogluconic acid. *Anal Biochem.* 1981;115:225–30.
3. Rose RC, Nahrwold DL. Quantitative analysis of ascorbic acid and dehydroascorbic acid by high-performance liquid chromatography. *Anal Biochem.* 1981;114:140–5.
4. Iwase H, Ono I. Determination of ascorbic acid and dehydroascorbic acid in juices by high-performance liquid chromatography with electrochemical detection using l-cysteine as precolumn reluctant. *J Chromatogr A.* 1993;654:215–20.
5. Lykkesfeldt J. Determination of ascorbic acid and dehydroascorbic acid in biological samples by high-performance liquid chromatography using subtraction methods: reliable reduction with tris[2-carboxyethyl]phosphine hydrochloride. *Anal Biochem.* 2000;282:89–93.

BILBERRY

Description

Botanical name: *Vaccinium myrtillus* L.

Common name: Whortleberry

Parts of plant used: Berries

Uses: To improve visual problems and circulatory disorders.

Mode of Action

About 20 clinical trials with bilberry have demonstrated positive effects for visual problems and circulatory disorders. The anthocyanins in bilberry are believed to be the bioactive components. The anthocyanins were found to have antioxidant, antiplatelet, anti-inflammatory, wound-healing, anti-ulcer, anti-atherosclerosis, ophthalmic, and vasoprotective activities. The anthocyanins also showed effects on vascular smooth muscle and arteriolar vasomotion. Also, the anthocyanins were found to interact with collagen, phospholipids, and proteoglycans.[1]

Chemical Markers

The chemical components of bilberry have been studied extensively. Several types of compounds including flavonoids, iridoids, organic acids, sugars, and terpenes have been found in bilberry. The several types of flavonoids found in bilberry include anthocyanins, flavonols, and flavan-3-ols. The ripe fruits were found to contain 5-hydroxylated anthocyanidins (delphinidin, cyanidin, petunidin, peonidin, malvidin), each of which is linked with three different sugar units, glucose, galactose, and arabinose. There are at least 15 anthocyanins in bilberry.

Bilberry is also well known to contain proanthocynidins, the amount of which decreases with the progression of ripening.[1,2] The volatile components of bilberry were also studied by GC and GC–MS methods; three compounds, *trans*-2-hexenal, ethyl 3-methylbutyrate, and ethyl 2-methylbutyrate were found to be responsible for the characteristic aroma of bilberry.[1] Currently in the U.S. market, anthocyanins are used as quality control standards for bilberry products.

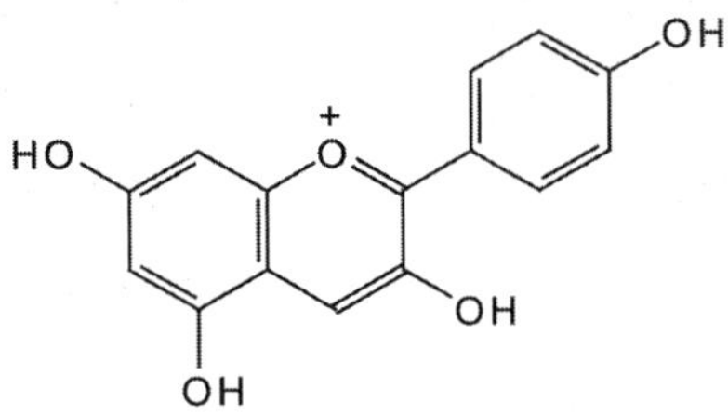

Pelargonidin

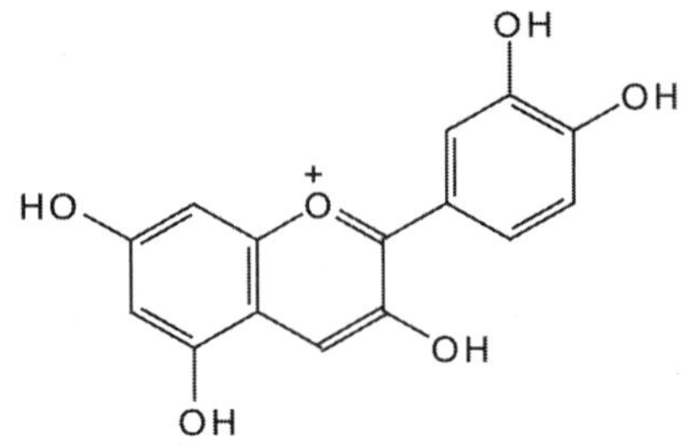

Cyanidin

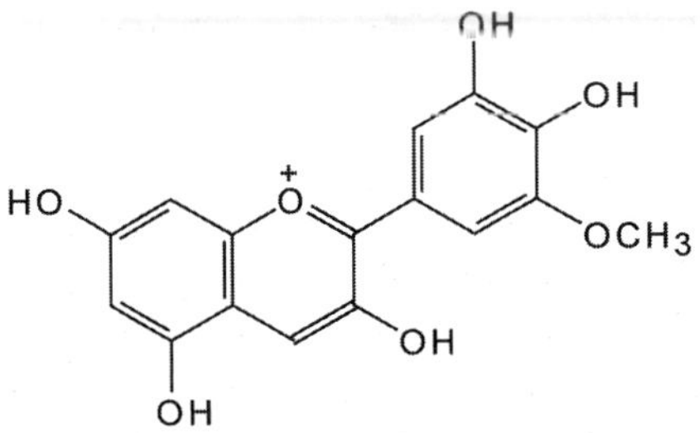

Petunidin

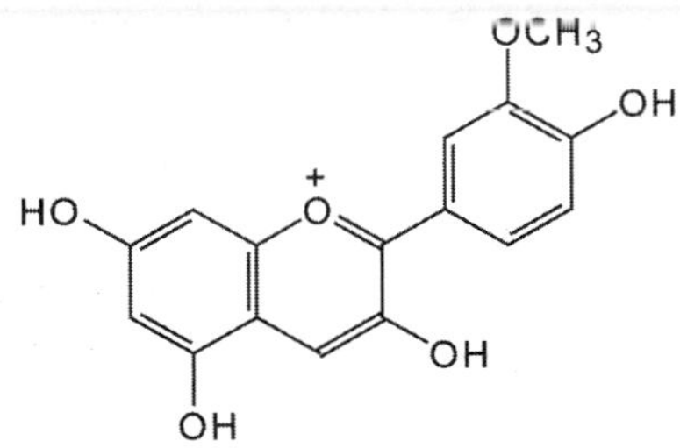

Peonidin

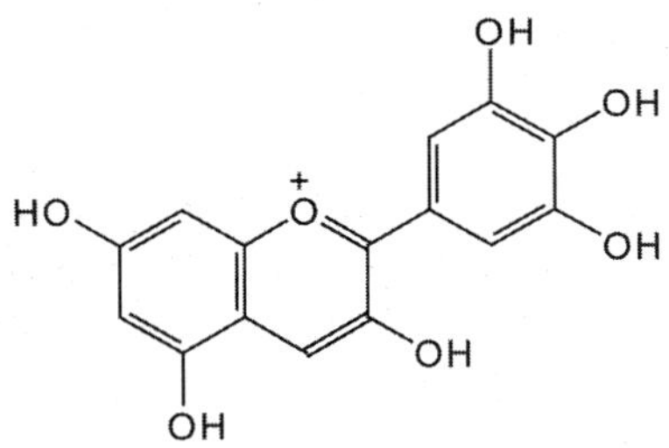

Delphinidin

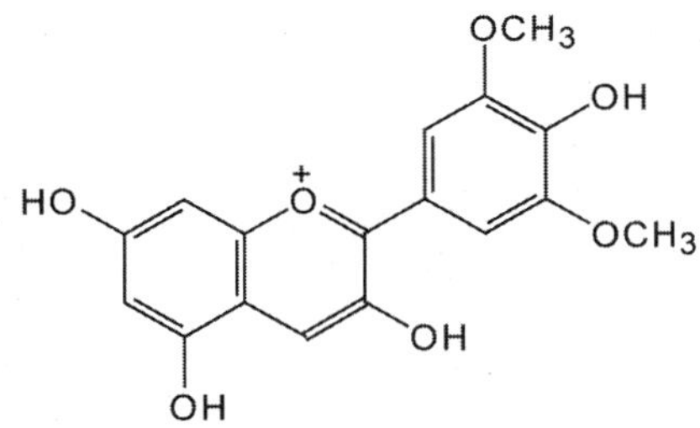

Malvidin

Methods of Analysis

Anthocyanins are usually analyzed by HPLC and colorimetric methods.

Method 1: The colorimetric method found at www.nsfina.org can be used to determine total anthocyanins in bilberry.

Preparation of buffers: To prepare the pH 1.0 buffer, dissolve 1.49 g of potassium chloride in 100 mL of deionized water, and then mix 25 mL of this solution with 67 mL of 0.2 N hydrochloric acid solution. Adjust the pH to 1.0±0.1 if necessary.

To prepare the pH 4.5 buffer, dissolve 1.64 g of sodium acetate in 100 mL of water and adjust the pH to 4.5±0.1 with hydrochloric acid.

Sample preparation: Weigh about 75 mg of powdered bilberry extract into a 100-mL volumetric flask and add about 80 mL of distilled water. Sonicate for 15 minutes or until dissolved. Cool to room temperature and dilute to volume with water. If the solution is not clear, centrifuge a portion to remove particulates. Dilute 1 mL of the bilberry solution to 25 mL with the pH 1.0 buffer and mix. And then dilute another 1 mL of the bilberry solution to 25 mL with the pH 4.5 buffer.

Testing: Zero the spectrophotometer with distilled water. Measure the absorbance of the pH 1.0 and 4.5 sample preparations at 510 and 700 nm, respectively.

Calculations: Calculate the difference in absorbance between the two samples using the following equation:

$$\text{Absorbance} = (A_{510nm}\ \text{pH } 1.0 - A_{700nm}\ \text{pH } 1.0) - (A_{510nm}\ \text{pH } 4.5 - A_{700nm}\ \text{pH } 4.5)$$

Calculate the %wt/wt of total anthocyanins in the sample using:

$$\%\text{wt/wt} = \text{Absorbance} \times \text{MW} \times \text{DF} \times \text{V} \times 100/(\varepsilon \times \text{L} \times \text{wt})$$

where:

A = absorbance
ε = Cyd-3-glu molar absorbance (26,900)
MW = anthocyanin molecular weight (449.2)
DF = dilution factor
V = final volume (mL)
wt = sample weight (mg)
L = cell pathlength (usually 1 cm)

Method 2: The method of Nyman and Kumpulainen[3] can be used to analyze the hydrolyzed aglycones of bilberry anthocyanins.

Sample preparation: Weigh about 0.5 g of dried sample into a 70-mL screw-cap test tube, add 18 to 60 mL of 2 M hydrochloric acid in methanol, and hydrolyze in a 90°C water bath for 50 minutes. Cool to room temperature and dilute to volume (25 to 100 mL) using methanol.

Chromatography

Column: Inertsil ODS3, 3 μm, 150 × 4.0 mm with a C18 guard column.

Mobile phase: Solvent A = water–formic acid (90:10), solvent B = acetonitrile.

Gradient:

Time (minutes)	%A	%B
0	96	4
8	85	15
23	85	15
24	20	80
27	20	80
28	96	4
34	96	4

Flow rate: 0.8 mL/minute

Injection volume: 10 μL

Detection wavelength: 530 nm for delphinidin, cyanidin, petunidin, peonidin, and malvidin, and 510 nm for pelargonidin.

Column temperature: 35°C

Validation data: Not available

Method 3: The method of Chandra et al.[4] can be used to identify the anthocyanins in bilberry.

Sample preparation: Not specified.

Chromatography

Column: Agilent Hypersil ODS, 5 μm, 125 × 4.0 mm.

Mobile phase: Solvent A = water (0.5% phosphoric acid), solvent B = water–acetonitrile–acetic acid–phosphoric acid (50:48.5:1.0:0.5 vol/vol/vol/vol).

Gradient: 20%B to 60%B in 26 minutes, then to 20%B in 4 minutes, and keep at 20%B for 5 minutes.

Flow rate: 0.8 mL/minute

Injection volume: 10 μL

Column temperature: 30°C

Detection wavelength: 520 nm

Validation data: Not available

Method 4: The method of Dugo et al.[5] was used.

Sample preparation: Pound about 200 g of fruit in a mortar to obtain the extract; centrifuge a 5-mL aliquot of extract at 6000 rpm for 20 minutes.

Chromatography

Column: Restek Pinnacle ODS, 5 μm, 250 × 4.6 mm.

Mobile phase: Solvent A = water–formic acid (9:1), solvent B = water–formic acid–acetonitrile (4:1:5).

Gradient: Hold at 12%B for 1 minute, then linear to 30%B in 25 minutes, and then to 100%B in 9 minutes.

Flow rate: 1 mL/minute

Injection volume: 20 μL

Detection wavelength: 518 nm

Validation data: Not available

References

1. Morazzoni P, Bombardelli E. *Vaccinium myrtillus* L. *Fitoterapia*. 1996;66(1):3–29.
2. Azar M, Verette E, Brun S. Identification of some phenolic compounds in bilberry juice *Vaccinium myrtillus*. *J Food Sci*. 1987;52(5):1255–7.
3. Nyman NA, Kumpulainen JT. Determination of anthocyanidins in berries and red wine by high-performance liquid chromatography. *J Agric Food Chem*. 2001;49(9):4183–7.
4. Chandra A, Rana J, Li Y. Separation, identification, quantification, and method validation of anthocyanins in botanical supplement raw materials by HPLC and HPLC–MS. *J Agric Food Chem*. 2001;49(8):3515–21.
5. Dugo P, Mondello L, Errante G, et al. Identification of anthocyanins in berries by narrow-bore high-performance liquid chromatography with electrospray ionization detection. *J Agric Food Chem*. 2001;49(8):3987–92.

BLACK COHOSH

Description

Botanical names: *Cimicifuga racemosa* (L.) Nutt.; *Actaea racemosa* L.

Common name: Black snakeroot

Parts of plant used: Dried rhizomes and roots

Uses: Treatment of symptoms of menopause, relief from premenstrual discomfort.

Mode of Action

Several clinical trials have proven the efficacy of black cohosh for menopausal symptoms. Earlier research found black cohosh improved neurovegetative symptoms and psychological complaints associated with hormonal deficiencies in women. The authors proposed that an estrogen-like effect was the primary mechanism of action. But current research shows that black cohosh's mode of action is not identical to estrogen and that black cohosh extract shows no estrogenic effects.[1]

Chemical Markers

Triterpene glycosides are the main chemical compounds in black cohosh root extract with 23-epi-26-deoxyactein (27-deoxyactein), actein, cimigenol-3-O-β-D-xylopyranoside, and cimiracemoside C (cimicifugoside M) as the main saponins. Recent research efforts have led to the isolation and identification of various novel triterpene glycosides:

Cimiracemosides A to P (Two new compounds named cimiracemoside A were reported in 2000. In the study of Shao et al.,[2] cimiracemoside A is 21-hydroxycimigenol-3-α-L-arabinopyranoside; in the paper by Bedir and Khan,[3] cimiracemoside A is 16β:23;22:25-diepoxy-12β-acetoxy-3β,23,24-trihydroxy-9,19-cycloanosta-7-ene-3-O-β-D-xylopyranoside, the same as cimiracemoside F in the Shao et al.[2] report.)

25-O-Methylcimigenol-3-O-α-L-arabinopyranoside (also named cimiracemoside B by Bedir and Khan,[3] but it is different from cimiracemoside B reported by Shao et al.[2]).

23-O-Acetylshengmanol-3-O-α-L-arabinopyranoside.

Shengmanol-3-O-β-L-arabinopyranoside.

25-O-Acetyl-12β-hydroxycimigenol-3-O-α-L-arabinopyranoside.

12β,21-Dihydroxycimigenol-3-O-α-L-arabinopyranoside.

(22R,23R,24R)-12β-Acetyloxy-16β:23;22:25-diepoxy-23,24-dihydroxy-9,19-cycloanosta-7-ene-3-O-α-L-arabinopyranoside.

Current research[2–9] also identified several known triterpene glycosides:

26-Deoxycimifugoside
25-O-Acetylshengmanol-3-O-β-D-xylopyranoside
Cimiaceroside A
12β-Hydroxycimigenol-3-O-β-D-xylopyranoside
12β-Hydroxycimigenol-3-O-α-L-arabinopyranoside
25-Anhydrocimigenol-3-O-β-D-xyloside
25-Anhydrocimigenol-3-O-α-L-arabinoside
25-O-Acetylcimigenol-3-O-β-D-xyloside
25-O-Acetylcimigenol-3-O-α-L-arabinoside
Cimicifugoside H-1
Cimicifugoside H-2
2′-Acetylacetein
25-O-Methylcimigenol-3-O-β-D-xylopyranoside

Phenolic compounds also were isolated from black cohosh. The isolated phenolic compounds include formononetin, kaempferol, isoferulic acid, ferulic acid, caffeic acid, methyl caffeate, fukinolic acid, cimicifugic acid A, cimicifugic acid B, cimicifugic acid F, and new compounds cimiracemate A to D.[10,11] Currently, the triterpene glycosides are used as marker compounds for quality control of black cohosh extract.

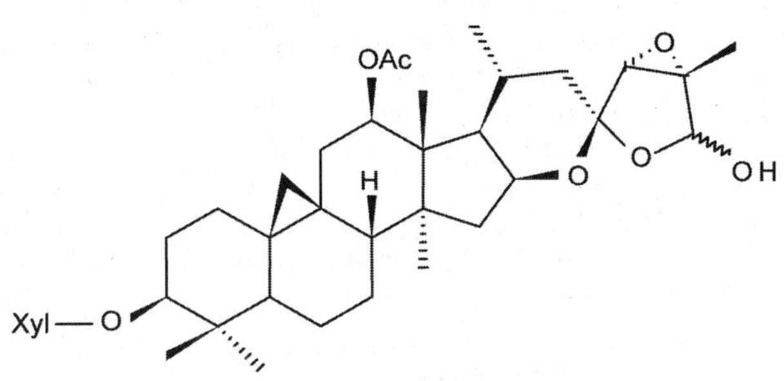

26-S and 26-R-Actein

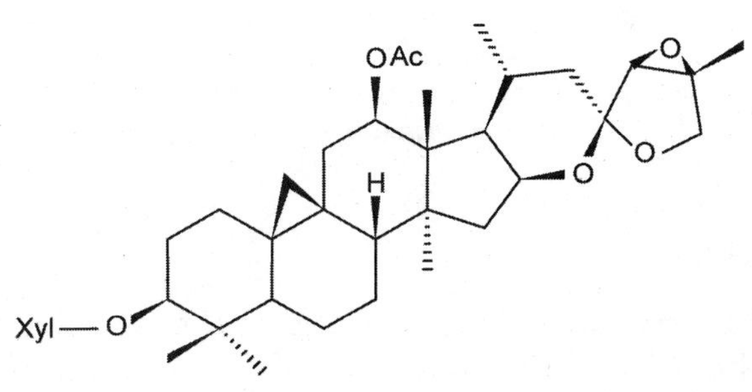

23-Epi-26-deoxyactein

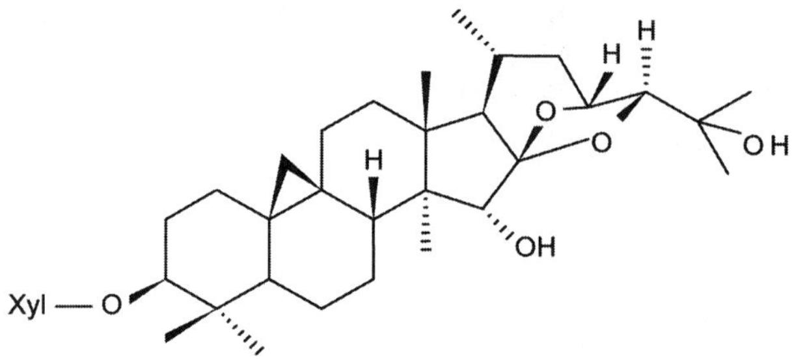

Cimigenol-3-xyloside

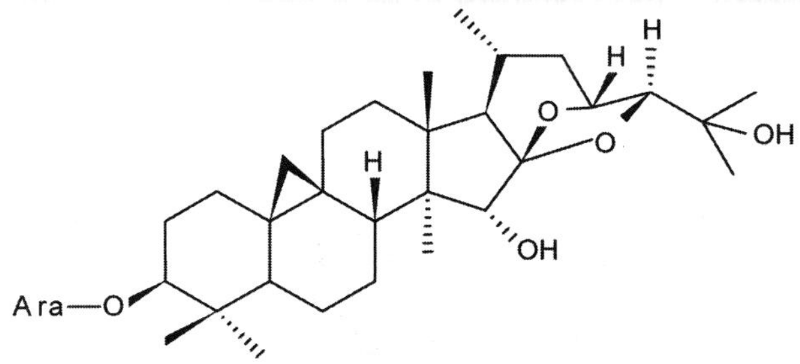

Cimiracemoside C (cimicifugoside M)

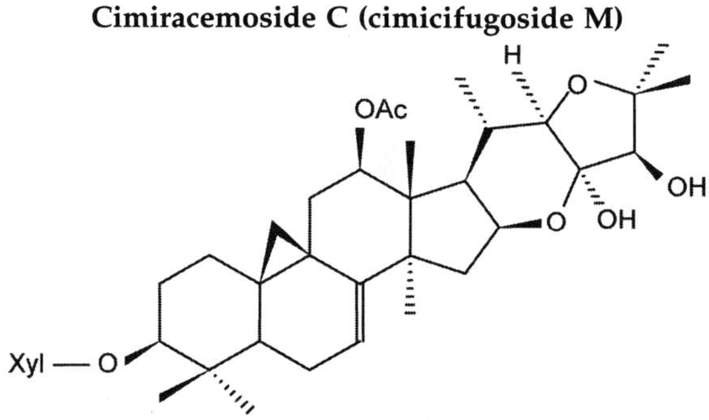

Cimiracemoside F

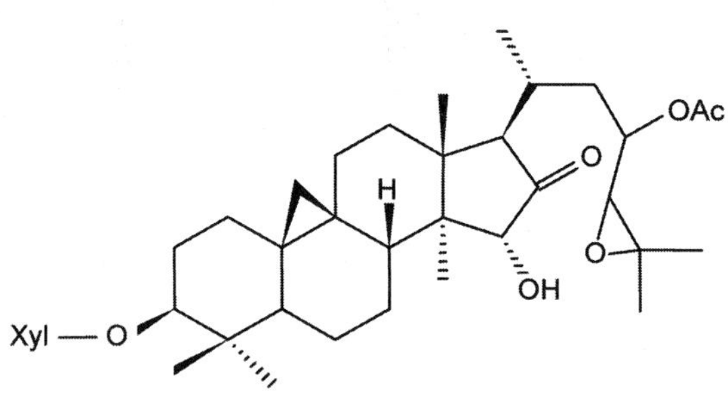

23-O-Acetylshengmanol-3-O-β-D-xyloside

Methods of Analysis

Several methods have been reported for the analysis of the triterpene glycosides in black cohosh, including HPLC coupled with an evaporative light-scattering detector (ELSD) or a MS detector.

Method 1: The method found at www.nsfina.org can be used to determine triterpene glycosides including actein, 26-deoxycimifugoside, cimiracemoside A, 26-deoxyactein, acetylshengmanolxyloside, cimicifugoside (cimigenol-3-O-β-D-xylopyranoside), cimiracemoside F, cimiracemoside C, and cimiracemoside E.

Sample preparation: For root material, mix 1.0 g of ground plant material with 40 mL of ethanol–water (50:50). Shake on an orbital or wrist-action shaker for 24 hours.

For the extract, sonicate 300 mg of powdered extract with 7 mL of methanol in a 10-mL volumetric flask for 30 minutes. Cool to room temperature and dilute to volume with methanol.

Chromatography

Column: Phenomenex Prodigy ODS3, 5 μm, 250 × 4.6 mm.
Mobile phase: Water (0.1% formic acid)–acetonitrile.
Gradient:

Time (minutes)	%A	%B
0	70	30
30	60	40
60	40	60
70	70	30

Column temperature: Room temperature (25°C)
Injection volume: 20 μL
Flow rate: 1.0 mL/minute
Detector: ELSD

Validation data: Not available, but this method is known to be a validated method.

Method 2: The method of Li et al.[12] can be used to analyze 16 compounds in black cohosh including caffeic acid, ferulic acid, isoferulic acid, cimicifugoside H-1, cimiracemoside F, cimicifugoside H-2, (26R)-actein, 26-deoxycimifugoside, (26S)-actein, 23-epi-26-deoxyactein, 23-O-acetylshengmanol-3-O-β-D-xyloside, 26-deoxyactein, 25-O-acetylshengmanol-3-O-α-L-arabinoside, 25-O-acetylshengmanol-3-O-β-D-xyloside, cimigenol-3-O-α-L-arabinoside (cimiracemoside C), and cimigenol-3-O-β-D-xyloside (cimicifugoside).

Sample preparation: For the liquid extract, directly filter the solution through a 0.22-μm membrane filter and use for HPLC analysis.

For the dried powdered extract, dissolve 30 mg in 1 mL of methanol using sonication.

For herbal powders, extract 0.5 to 1.0 g of sample with 15 mL of methanol twice using sonication for 30 minutes. Combine the methanol extracts and evaporate to dryness under reduced pressure. Dissolve the residue in 10 mL of methanol.

For commercial dietary supplements, extract one dosage unit of the product with 25 mL of methanol (100% methanol for capsules, 80% methanol for caplets, and 50% methanol for tablets) twice using sonication for 30 minutes. Combine the methanol extracts and use for HPLC analysis.

Chromatography

Column: Waters YMC ODS-AQ RP18, 250 × 4.6 mm, 5 μm with a Waters Delta-Pak RP18 guard column, 5 × 4.6 mm.

Mobile phase: Solvent A = water (0.05% trifluoroacetic acid), solvent B = acetonitrile.

Gradient:

Time (minutes)	%A	%B
0	80	20
8	80	20
15	68	32
55	36	64
65	5	95
70	5	95

Flow rate: 1.6 mL/minute

Injection volume: 10 μL

Detection wavelength: ELSD detector

Validation data:

Linearity: 10 to 100 mcg/mL for caffeic acid, ferulic acid, and isoferulic acid, 10 to 340 mcg/mL for cimicifugoside H-2, 11 to 110 mcg/mL for cimiracemoside F, 10 to 340 mcg/mL for cimicifugoside H-2, 3.5 to 12 mcg/mL for (26R)-actein, 5.3 to 53 mcg/mL for 26-deoxycimifugoside, 8 to 80 mcg/mL for (26S)-actein, 10 to 320 mcg/mL for 23-epi-26-deoxyactein, 9 to 90 mcg/mL for 23-O-acetylshengmanol-3-O-β-D-xyloside, 10 to 100 mcg/mL for 26-deoxyactein, 9 to 90 mcg/mL for 25-O-acetylshengmanol-3-O-α-L-arabinoside, 10 to 100 mcg/mL for 25-O-acetylshengmanol-3-O-β-D-xyloside, 6.5 to 125 mcg/mL for cimigenol-3-O-α-L-arabinoside (cimiracemoside C), and 6.5 to 65 mcg/mL for cimigenol-3-O-β-D-xyloside (cimicifugoside). The correlation coefficients were more than 0.9949 for all compounds.

Accuracy: The percent recoveries were from 91.75 to 99.96 for six selected compounds.

Precision: Not specified

Selectivity: Peak identification was determined against standards.

Ruggedness: Not specified

Robustness: Not specified

LOD/LOQ: LOD = 24 to 53 ng for all 16 standards.

References

1. Liske E, Hanggi W, Henneicke-von Zepelin HH, et al. Physiological investigation of a unique extract of black cohosh (*Cimicifugae racemosae* rhizoma): a 6-month clinical study demonstrates no systemic estrogenic effect. *J Womens Health Gend Based Med.* 2002;11(2):163–74.
2. Shao Y, Harris A, Wang M, et al. Triterpene glycosides from *Cimicifuga racemosa. J Nat Prod.* 2000;63(7):905–10.
3. Bedir E, Khan IA. Cimiracemoside A: a new cyclolanostanol xyloside from the rhizome of *Cimicifuga racemosa. Chem Pharm Bull.* 2000;48(3):425–7.
4. Chen SN, Fabricant DS, Lu ZZ, et al. Cimiracemosides I-P, new 9,19-cyclolanostane triterpene glycosides from *Cimicifuga racemosa. J Nat Prod.* 2002;65(10):1391–7.
5. Chen SN, Li W, Fabricant DS, et al. Isolation, structure elucidation, and absolute configuration of 26-deoxyactein from *Cimicifuga racemosa* and clarification of nomenclature associated with 27-deoxyactein. *J Nat Prod.* 2002;65(4):601–5.
6. Watanabe K, Mimaki Y, Sakagami H, et al. Cycloartane glycosides from the rhizomes of *Cimicifuga racemosa* and their cytotoxic activities. *Chem Pharm Bull.* 2002;50(1):121–5.
7. Bedir E, Khan IA. A new cyclolanostanol arabinoside from the rhizome of *Cimicifuga racemosa. Pharmazie.* 2001;56(3):268–9.
8. Hamburger M, Wegner C, Benthin B. Cycloartane glycosides from *Cimicifuga racemosa. Pharm Pharmacol Lett.* 2001;11(2):98–100.
9. He K, Zheng B, Kim CH, et al. Direct analysis and identification of triterpene glycosides by LC/MS in black cohosh, *Cimicifuga racemosa,* and in several commercially available black cohosh products. *Planta Med.* 2000;66(7):635–40.
10. Chen SN, Fabricant DS, Lu ZZ, et al. Cimiracemates A-D, phenylpropanoid esters from the rhizomes of *Cimicifuga racemosa. Phytochemistry.* 2002;61(4):409–13.
11. Burdette JE, Chen SN, Lu ZZ, et al. Black cohosh (*Cimicifuga racemosa* L.) protects against menadione-induced DNA damage through scavenging of reactive oxygen species: bioassay-directed isolation and characterization of active principles. *J Agric Food Chem.* 2002;50(24):7022–8.
12. Li W, Chen S, Fabricant D, et al. High-performance liquid chromatographic analysis of black cohosh (*Cimicifuga racemosa*) constituents with in-line evaporative light scattering and photodiode array detection. *Anal Chim Acta.* 2002;471(1):61–75.

BOSWELLIA

Description

Botanical name: *Boswellia serrata*

Common names: Boswellin, Indian frankincense

Parts of plant used: Gum resin

Uses: Treatment of inflammatory and arthritic disease; as anticancer agent.

Mode of Action

Promising results were found in clinical trials in patients with bronchial asthma, chronic colitis, Crohn's disease, osteoarthritis of the knee, rheumatoid arthritis, and ulcerative colitis.[1–5] The pentacyclic triterpene acids, namely boswellic acids, in the gum resin are believed to be the anti-inflammatory components. Boswellic acids were found to suppress leukotriene synthesis via inhibition of 5-lipoxygenase, which was considered as the main mechanism for its anti-inflammatory activity.[6–8] Recently, the gum was found to be an anticancer agent and to trigger apoptosis.[9–14]

Chemical Markers

Boswellic acid-type pentacyclic triterpene acids are the major components in boswellia gum; the identified boswellic acids include α-boswellic acid, β-boswellic acid, 11-keto-β-boswellic acid, 3-α-acetyl-11-keto-β-boswellic acid, 3-acetyl-α-boswellic acid, 3-acetyl-β-boswellic acid, 3-α-acetyl-20(29)-lupene-24-oic acid, 3-α-acetyl-9,11-dehydrox-β-boswellic acid, and 3-α-acetyl-9,11-dehydro-α-boswellic acid.[15–18]

Other compounds purified from boswellia gum included tetracyclic triterpenes, diterpene (serratol), and saponins.[19–21] The essential oil from gum was found to contain d-α-thujene and p-cymene as the main components. Other minor compounds (β-pinene, d-limonene, linalool, terpineol, methylchavicol, terpinyl acetate, cadinene, geraniol, and elemol) were also isolated from the oil.[22] As the boswellic acids are the bioactive components in *Boswellia,* they are used as marker compounds for quality control of boswellic gum; usually, six boswellic acids are analyzed: α-boswellic acid, β-boswellic acid, 11-keto-β-boswellic acid, 3-α-acetyl-11-keto-β-boswellic acid, 3-acetyl-α-boswellic acid, and 3-acetyl-β-boswellic acid.

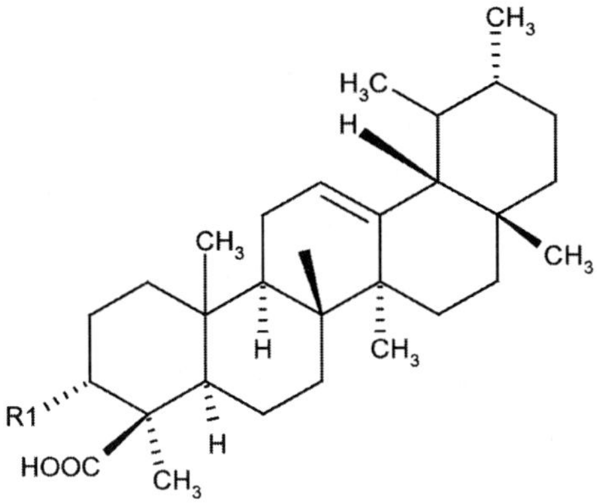

β-Boswellic acid: R_1 = OH
3-Acetyl-β-boswellic acid: R_1 = OAc

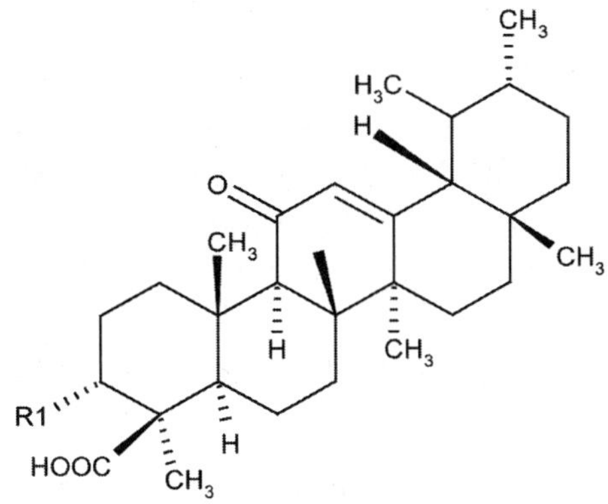

11-Keto-β-boswellic acid: R_1 = OH
3-Acetyl-11-keto-β-boswellic acid: R_1 = OAc

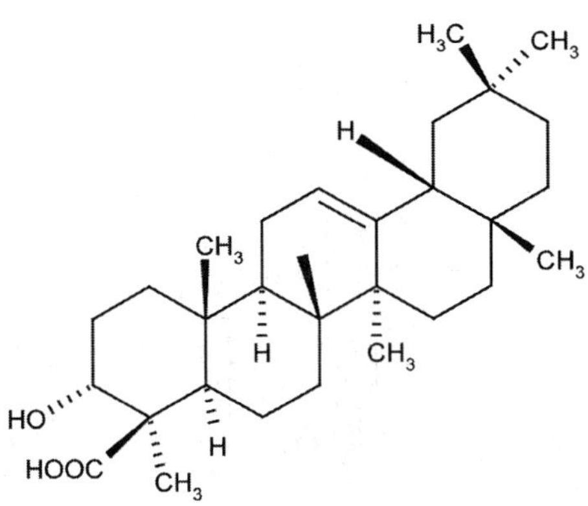

α-Boswellic acid

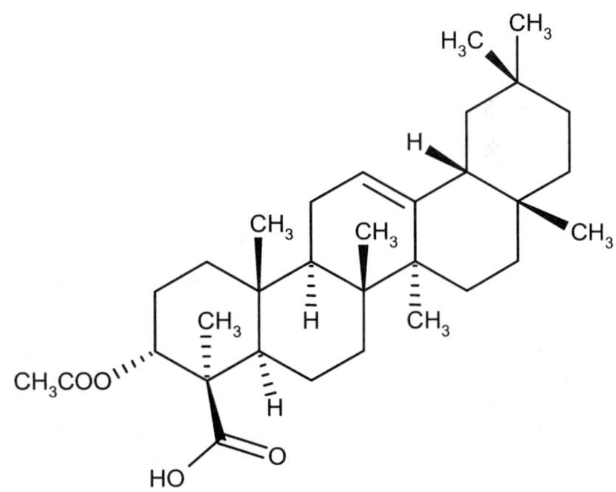

3-Acetyl-α-boswellic acid

Major boswellic acids in *Boswellia*.

Methods of Analysis

Very few methods have been officially published for analysis of *Boswellia.* One accepted HPLC method and several TLC methods have been published for analysis of boswellic acid content in boswellia gum.[18,23,24]

Method 1: The HPLC method of Ganzera and Khan[18] can be used to analyze six boswellic acids: α-boswellic acid, β-boswellic acid, 11-keto-β-boswellic acid, 3-α-acetyl-11-keto-β-boswellic acid, 3-acetyl-α-boswellic acid, and 3-acetyl-β-boswellic acid.

Sample preparation: Sonicate 100 mg of pure resin or 500 mg of market product in 3 mL of methanol for 10 minutes. Centrifuge and take out the supernates, and repeat the procedures two times. Transfer the supernates to a 10-mL volumetric flask and dilute to 10 mL with methanol.

Chromatography

Column: Phenomenex Synergi MAX-RP-80 A, 4 µm, 150 × 4.6 mm.

Mobile phase: Solvent A = water (containing 0.05% phosphoric acid), solvent B = acetonitrile (containing 0.05% phosphoric acid).

Gradient: 0 to 7 minutes isocratic 35%A and 65%B, then in 28 minutes to 10%A and 90%B and keep this composition for 5 more minutes. Follow by 100%B washing for 5 minutes.

Flow rate: 1.0 mL/minute

Injection volume: 10 µL

Detection wavelength: 210 nm

Column temperature: 60°C

Validation data:

Linearity: 8 to 500 mcg/mL with a correlation coefficient of 0.999 for all six compounds.

Accuracy: The percent recovery was between 97.2 and 100.1 for six marker compounds.

Precision: Maximum RSD was 3.28%.

Selectivity: Peak identification was determined against standards.

Ruggedness: Not specified

Robustness: Not specified

LOD/LOQ: The limit of detection was at least 0.90 mcg/mL or lower.

References

1. Ammon HP. Boswellic acids (components of frankincense) as the active principle in treatment of chronic inflammatory diseases. *Wien Med Wochenschr.* 2002;152(15–16):373–8.
2. Kimmatkar N, Thawani V, Hingorani L, et al. Efficacy and tolerability of *Boswellia serrata* extract in treatment of osteoarthritis of knee—a randomized double-blind placebo-controlled trial. *Phytomedicine.* 2003;10(1):3–7.
3. Gupta I, Parihar A, Malhotra P, et al. Effects of gum resin of *Boswellia serrata* in patients with chronic colitis. *Planta Med.* 2001;67(5):391–5.
4. Gupta I, Gupta V, Parihar A, et al. Effects of *Boswellia serrata* gum resin in patients with bronchial asthma: results of a double-blind, placebo-controlled, 6-week clinical study. *Eur J Med Res.* 1998;3(11):511–4.
5. Gupta I, Parihar A, Malhotra P, et al. Effects of *Boswellia serrata* gum resin in patients with ulcerative colitis. *Eur J Med Res.* 1997;2(1):37–43.
6. Safayhi H, Boden SE, Schweizer S, et al. Concentration-dependent potentiating and inhibitory effects of Boswellia extracts on 5-lipoxygenase product formation in stimulated PMNL. *Planta Med.* 2000;66(2):110–3.
7. Safayhi H, Sailer ER, Ammon HP. 5-Lipoxygenase inhibition by acetyl-11-keto-β-boswellic acid (AKBA) by a novel mechanism. *Phytomedicine.* 1996;3(1):71–2.
8. Ammon HP, Safayhi H, Mack T, et al. Mechanism of antiinflammatory actions of curcumine and boswellic acids. *J Ethnopharmacol.* 1993;38(2–3):113–9.

9. Liu JJ, Nilsson A, Oredsson S, et al. Boswellic acids trigger apoptosis via a pathway dependent on caspase-8 activation but independent on Fas/Fas ligand interaction in colon cancer HT-29 cells. *Carcinogenesis.* 2002;23(12):2087–93.
10. Hostanska K, Daum G, Saller R. Cytostatic and apoptosis-inducing activity of boswellic acids toward malignant cell lines in vitro. *Anticancer Res.* 2002;22(5):2853–62.
11. Liu JJ, Nilsson A, Oredsson S, et al. Keto- and acetyl-keto-boswellic acids inhibit proliferation and induce apoptosis in Hep G2 cells via a caspase-8 dependent pathway. *Int J Mol Med.* 2002;10(4):501–5.
12. Park YS, Lee JH, Bondar J, et al. Cytotoxic action of acetyl-11-keto-β-boswellic acid (AKBA) on meningioma cells. *Planta Med.* 2002;68(5):397–401.
13. Huang MT, Badmaev V, Ding Y, et al. Anti-tumor and anti-carcinogenic activities of triterpenoid, β-boswellic acid. *BioFactors.* 2000;13(1–4):225–30.
14. Shao Y, Ho CT, Chin CK, et al. Inhibitory activity of boswellic acids from *Boswellia serrata* against human leukemia HL-60 cells in culture. *Planta Med.* 1998;64(4):328–31.
15. Belsner K, Buchele B, Werz U, et al. Structural analysis of pentacyclic triterpenes from the gum resin of *Boswellia serrata* by NMR spectroscopy. *Magn Reson Chem.* 2003;41(2):115–22.
16. Belsner K, Buchele B, Werz U, et al. Structural analysis of 3-α-acetyl-20(29)-lupene-24-oic acid, a novel pentacyclic triterpene isolated from the gum resin of *Boswellia serrata,* by NMR spectroscopy. *Magn Reson Chem.* 2003;41(8):629–32.
17. Pardhy RS, Bhattacharyya SC. β-Boswellic acid, acetyl-β-boswellic acid, acetyl-11-keto-β-boswellic acid and 11-keto-β-boswellic acid, four pentacyclic triterpene acids from the resin of *Boswellia serrata* Roxb. *Ind J Chem.* 1978;16B(3):176–8.
18. Ganzera M, Khan IA. A reversed-phase high-performance liquid chromatography method for the analysis of boswellic acids in *Boswellia serrata. Planta Med.* 2001;67(8):778–80.
19. Pardhy RS, Bhattacharyya SC. Tetracyclic triterpene acids from the resin of *Boswellia serrata* Roxb. *Ind J Chem.* 1978;16B(3):174–5.
20. Pardhy RS, Bhattacharyya SC. Structure of serratol, a new diterpene cembranoid alcohol from *Boswellia serrata* Roxb. *Ind J Chem.* 1978;16B(3):171–3.
21. Gangwal ML, Vardhan DK. Stigmasta-5,24(28)-diene saponin from *Boswellia serrata. Ultra Scientist of Physical Sciences.* 1995;7(1):108–9.
22. Girgune JB, Garg BD. Chemical investigation of the essential oil from *Boswellia serrata* Roxb. *J Sci Res.* 1979;1(3):119–22.
23. Krohn K, Rao MS, Raman NV, et al. High-performance thin layer chromatographic analysis of anti-inflammatory triterpenoids from *Boswellia serrata* Roxb. *Phytochem Anal.* 2001;12(6):374–6.
24. Sane RT, Phadke MM, Hijli PS, et al. A high performance thin layer chromatography method for the simultaneous quantitative analysis of gugul (*Boswellia serrata*) and turmeric (*Curcuma longa*) from an ayurvedic preparation. *Indian Drugs.* 1998;35(5):286–90.

CHAMOMILE

Description

Botanical names: *Matricaria recutita* L.; *Chamomilla recutita* (L.) Rausch; *Matricaria chamomilla* L.

Common names: German chamomile, Hungarian chamomile

Parts of plant used: Flowering tops, flowers

Uses: As an antispasmodic, anti-inflammatory, or sedative.

Mode of Action

Several clinical trials have been performed on chamomile, and this herb has been proven effective for treating respiratory, neurological, and dermatological conditions. The apigenin-type flavonoids and the volatile oil components (chamazulene and α-bisabolol) were found to be responsible in part for its activity.

Chemical Markers

Chamomile is well known to contain flavonoids, coumarins, sesquiterpenoid lactones, and phenolic acids. Apigenin, apigenin-7-glucoside and its acetylated derivatives (2″-, 3″-, 4″-, 6″-monoacetates and 2″,3″-, 3″,4″-diacetates) were found to be the major flavonoids in the flowers; other flavonoids include luteolin glycosides, quercetin glycosides, and isorhamnetin glycosides.[1,2] Chamomile also contains 0.3% to 1.5% oils. The major oil constituents were bisabolol oxide A and B, chamazulene, spiroether, farnesene, and spathulenol.[3] Chamomile oil usually has a blue color, owing to chamazulene, which is produced from decomposition of the sesquiterpenoid lactone matricin.[1] Apigenin and apigenin-7-glucoside are related flavonoids used as marker compounds for quality control of chamomile extracts.

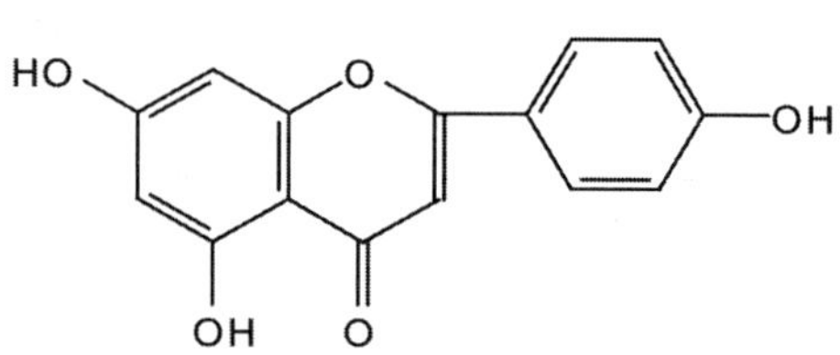

Apigenin

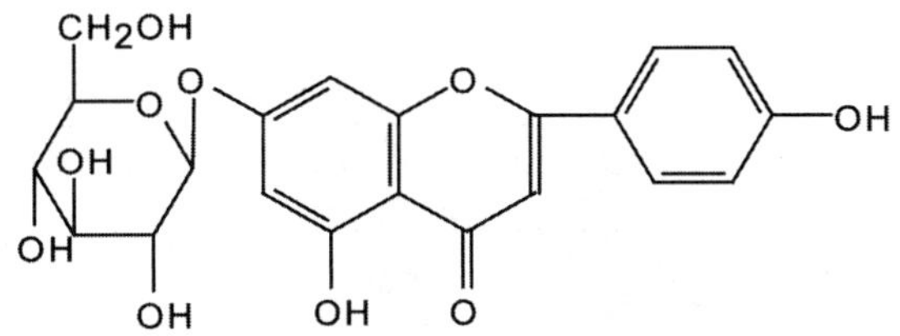

Apigenin-7-glucoside

Methods of Analysis

Apigenin-types flavonoids are usually analyzed by HPLC because of their strong UV absorptions.

Method 1: The method of Repcak and Martonfi[2] was used.

Sample preparation: Extract the sample with methanol.

Chromatography

Column: SGX C18, 7 µm, 150 × 3.0 mm.

Mobile phase: Solvent A = acetonitrile–water–phosphoric acid (19:40:1), solvent B = acetonitrile–methanol–phosphoric acid (59:40:1).

Gradient:

Time (minutes)	%A	%B
0	76	24
5	70	30
10	62	38
15	46	54
21	30	70
25	15	85
30	76	24

Flow rate: 1 mL/minute

Injection volume: 20 µL

Detection wavelength: 335 nm

Validation data: Not available

Method 2: The method of Redaelli et al.[4] was used.

Sample preparation: Reflux 100 to 120 mg of sample with 80 mL of methanol for 1 hour. Filter, concentrate the extraction solution, and adjust to volume (10 mL).

Chromatography

Column: PerkinElmer HC–ODS Sil-X reversed-phase, 150 × 4.6 mm.

Mobile phase: Solvent A = acetonitrile–water–acetic acid (15:83:2), solvent B = acetonitrile–water–acetic acid (60:38:2).

Gradient: A to B in 25 minutes.

Injection volume: 5 µL

Detection wavelength: 335 nm

Flow rate: 1 mL/minute

Validation data: Not available

Method 3: The method of Schulz and Albroscheit[5] was used.

Sample preparation: Dissolve about 150 mg of plant extract in 5 mL of distilled water and load the solution onto a 3-mL Bakerbond C18 SPE cartridge, first washed by 30 mL of distilled water, then washed by 10 mL of methanol containing 0.2 mL of 25% ammonia solution. Evaporate the methanol solution to dryness and dissolve in 1 mL of methanol.

Chromatography

Column: Hewlett-Packard Hypersil ODS microbore, 5 µm, 100 × 2.1 mm.

Mobile phase: Solvent A = water (adjusted to pH 2.8 with phosphoric acid), solvent B = acetonitrile.

Gradient:

Time (minutes)	%A	%B
0	97.5	2.5
9.9	97.5	2.5
10	80	20
14.9	80	20
15	65	35
16.9	65	35
17	0	100
20	0	100

Detection wavelength: 337 nm

Flow rate: 0.5 mL/minute

Injection volume: 2 to 10 µL

Column temperature: 40°C

References

1. Bruneton J. *Pharmacognosy, Phytochemistry, Medicinal Plants.* Paris: Lavoisier Publishing; 1995:455–7.
2. Repcak M, Martonfi P. The variability pattern of apigenin glucosides in *Chamomilla recutita* diploid and tetraploid cultivars. *Pharmazie.* 1995;50:696–9.
3. Weglarz Z, Roslon W. Individual variability of chamomile [*Chamomilla recutita* (L.) Rausch.] in respect of the content and chemical composition of essential oil. *Herba Polonica.* 2002;48(4):169–73.
4. Redaelli C, Formentini L, Santaniello E. Reversed-phase high-performance liquid chromatography analysis of apigenin and its glucosides in flowers of *Matricaria chamomilla* and chamomile extracts. *Planta Med.* 1981;42:293–5.
5. Schulz H, Albroscheit G. High-performance liquid chromatographic characterization of some medical plant extracts used in cosmetic formulas. *J Chromatogr A.* 1988;442:353–61.

CHASTE TREE

Description

Botanical name: *Vitex agnus-castus* L.

Common names: Agnus-castus, Monk's pepper, vitex

Parts of plant used: Berries

Uses: Relief of premenstrual syndrome and painful menstruation; treatment of corpus luteum insufficiency.

Mode of Action

Several clinical trials have demonstrated positive effects of chaste tree for treating corpus luteum abnormalities, premenstrual syndrome, and menstrual cycle abnormalities. However, the compounds responsible for chaste tree berry's activities are unknown, although some diterpenes showed dopaminergic properties and were found to bind to recombinant DA2-receptor protein and to suppress prolactin release, which may result in improving premenstrual mastodynia and possibly other symptoms of the premenstrual syndrome.[1–3]

Chemical Markers

Several groups of natural products have been identified in chaste tree berries including flavonoids with casticin as the major lipophilic flavone, iridoid glycosides with agnuside as the major one, diterpenes such as rotundifuran, vitexilactone, vitetrifolin D, and vitexlactum A.[4–6] Other compounds purified from flowering tops and root barks of chaste tree include agnucastoside A, B, and C; mussaenosidic acid; 6′-O-p-hydroxybenzoylmussaenosidic acid; myzodendrone; luteolin 6-C-(4″-methyl-6″-O-*trans*-caffeoylglucoside); luteolin-6-C-(6″-*trans*-caffeoylglucoside); luteolin 7-O-(6″-p-benzoylglucoside); luteolin; artemetin; and isorhamnetin.[7,8] Dried chaste tree berries also contain 0.15% to 1% essential oil with sabinene, 1,8-cineole, (E)-β-farnesene, α-pinene, and β-caryophylene as the major volatiles.[9] Currently in the market, casticin and agnuside are used as marker compounds for quality control of chaste tree berries.

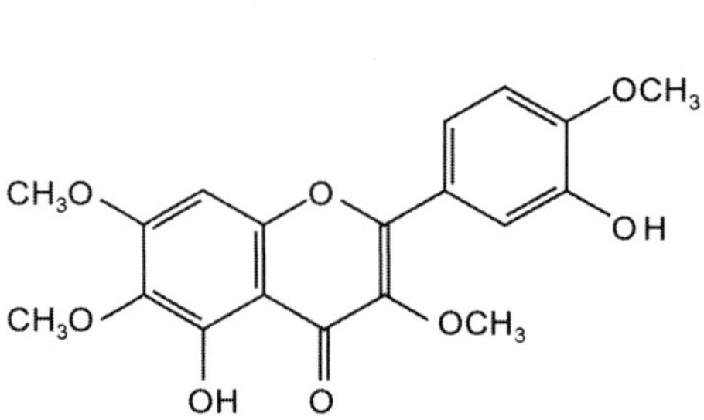

Casticin

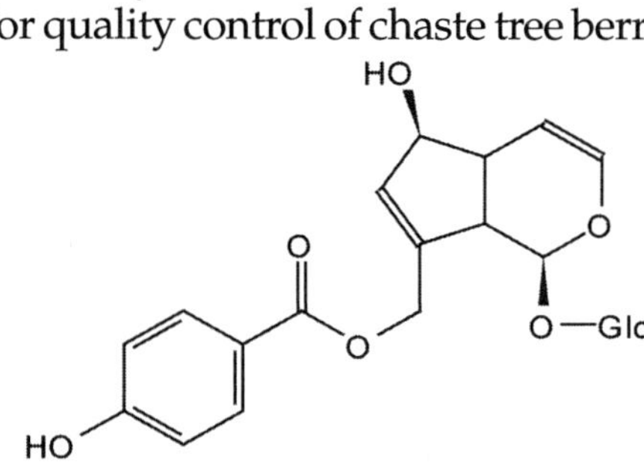

Agnuside

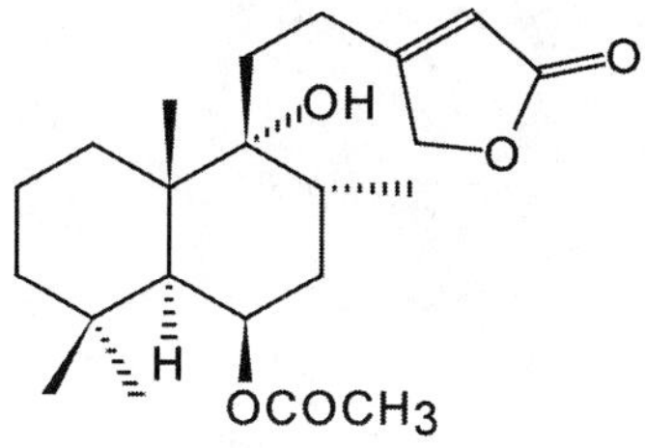

Vitexilactone

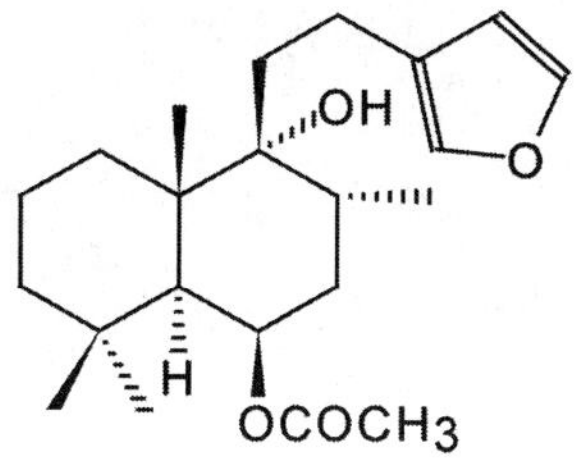

Rotundifuran

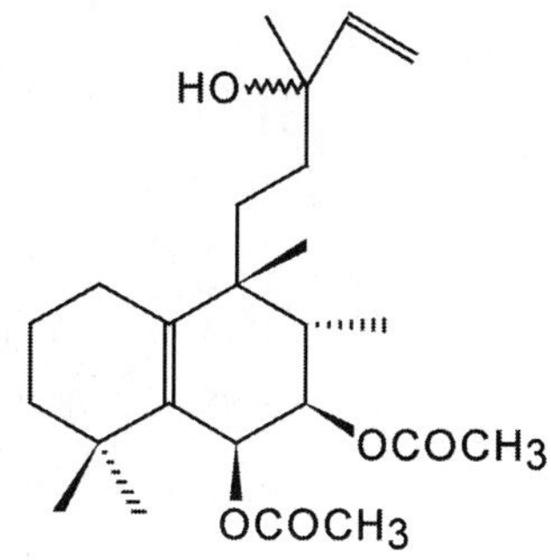

Vitetrifolin D

Methods of Analysis

HPLC is the most accepted method for quality control of chaste tree extract. Several HPLC methods have been developed to analyze casticin, agnuside, and diterpenes in the berries.

Method 1: The method of Hoberg et al.[10] can be used for the analysis of casticin.

Sample preparation: Extract 1 g of sample twice by turbo extraction at 19,000 rpm with 40 mL of methanol for 2 minutes. Rinse the residues using a small amount of methanol. Combine the resulting solutions, evaporate to dryness, and dissolve the residue in 20 mL of methanol.

Chromatography

Column: Hypersil ODS, 5 µm, 125 × 3.1 mm.

Mobile phase: Solvent A = water (0.5% phosphoric acid), solvent B = methanol.

Gradient:

Time (minutes)	%A	%B
0	50	50
13	35	65
13.1	0	100
18	0	100
18.1	50	50
25	50	50

Flow rate: 1.0 mL/minute

Injection volume: 10 µL

Detection wavelength: 258 nm

Column temperature: 25°C

Validation data:

Linearity: 25 to 125 mcg/mL with a correlation coefficient of 0.996.

Accuracy: The extract was spiked with 30%, 50%, and 80% of the expected amount of casticin; the percent recovery was 98.2 (2.2% RSD).

Precision: 2.6% RSD (six determinations)

Selectivity: Peak identification was determined against standards.

Ruggedness: Not specified

Robustness: Not specified

LOD/LOQ: Not specified

Method 2: The method of Hoberg et al.[11] was used for the determination of agnuside.

Sample preparation: Extract 1 g of sample twice by turbo extraction at 19,000 rpm with 40 mL of methanol for 2 minutes. Rinse the residues using a small amount of methanol. Combine the resulting solutions and evaporate to dryness. Dissolve the residue in 2 mL of water–methanol (95:5) and subject this solution to solid-phase extraction over neutral aluminum oxide. Adjust the final solution volume to 10 mL with water–methanol (95:5).

Chromatography

Column: Hypersil ODS, 5 μm, 125 × 3.1 mm.

Mobile phase: Solvent A = water (0.5% phosphoric acid), solvent B = acetonitrile.

Gradient:

Time (minutes)	%A	%B
0	93	7
0.6	90	10
5	90	10
7	86	14
13	85	15
13.1	0	100
18	0	100
18.1	93	7
23	93	7

Flow rate: 1.3 mL/minute

Injection volume: 10 μL

Detection wavelength: 258 nm

Column temperature: 25°C

Validation data:

Linearity: 1.3 to 422 mcg/mL with a correlation coefficient of 0.9998.

Accuracy: The extract was spiked with 30%, 50%, and 80% of the expected amount of casticin; the percent recovery was 98.3.

Precision: 3.22% RSD (six determinations)

Selectivity: Peak identification was determined against standards.

Ruggedness: Not specified

Robustness: Not specified

LOD/LOQ: Not specified

Method 3: The method of Hoberg et al.[11] was used for the determination of diterpenes, rotundifuran, vitexilactone, and 6β,7β-diacetoxy-13-hydroxy-labda-8,14-diene (later on this compound was corrected to vitetrifolin D).

Sample preparation: For fruit powders, extract 1 g of fruits twice by turbo extraction at 19,000 rpm with 40 mL of methanol for 2 minutes, and rinse the residues using a small amount of methanol. Combine the resulting solutions and evaporate to dryness. Dissolve the residue in 10 mL of acetonitrile–water (4:1).

For extracts, dissolve 0.2 g of extract in 10 mL of acetonitrile–water (4:1).

Chromatography

Column: Hypersil ODS, 5 μm, 125 × 3.1 mm.

Mobile phase: Solvent A = water, solvent B = acetonitrile.

Gradient:

Time (minutes)	%A	%B
0	60	40
5	52	48
30	52	48
30.01	0	100
35	0	100
35.01	60	40
45	60	40

Flow rate: 1.0 mL/minute

Injection volume: 20 μL

Detection wavelength: 210 nm

Column temperature: 25°C

Validation data:

Linearity: 31 to 155, 26 to 130, and 52 to 260 mcg/mL for vitexilactone, vitetrifolin D, and rotundifuran, respectively, with correlation coefficients greater than 0.996.

Accuracy: The percent recoveries were 105, 103, and 100 for vitexilactone, vitetrifolin D, and rotundifuran, respectively.

Precision: RSD was less than 3.4% for three compounds (six determinations).

Selectivity: Peak identification was determined against standards.

Ruggedness: Not specified

Robustness: Not specified

LOD: 1.3 mcg for rotundifuran, 0.325 mcg for vitetrifolin D, and 0.069 mcg for vitexilactone.

Method 4: The unpublished method of Mingfu Wang was used for the determination of agnuside.

Sample preparation: Weigh 400 mg of extract into a 50-mL volumetric flask. Add 35 mL of 70% methanol aqueous solution. Sonicate the sample for 30 minutes. Cool to room temperature and dilute to volume with 70% methanol.

Chromatography

Column: Phenomenex Luna C18(2), 5 μm, 250 × 4.6 mm.

Mobile phase: Solvent A = water (0.1% phosphoric acid), solvent B = acetonitrile

Gradient:

Time (minutes)	%A	%B
0	90	10
10	80	20
15	70	30
20	50	50
21	90	10
30	90	10

Flow rate: 1 mL/minute

Detector: 258 nm

Injection volume: 10 μL

Validation data: Not available

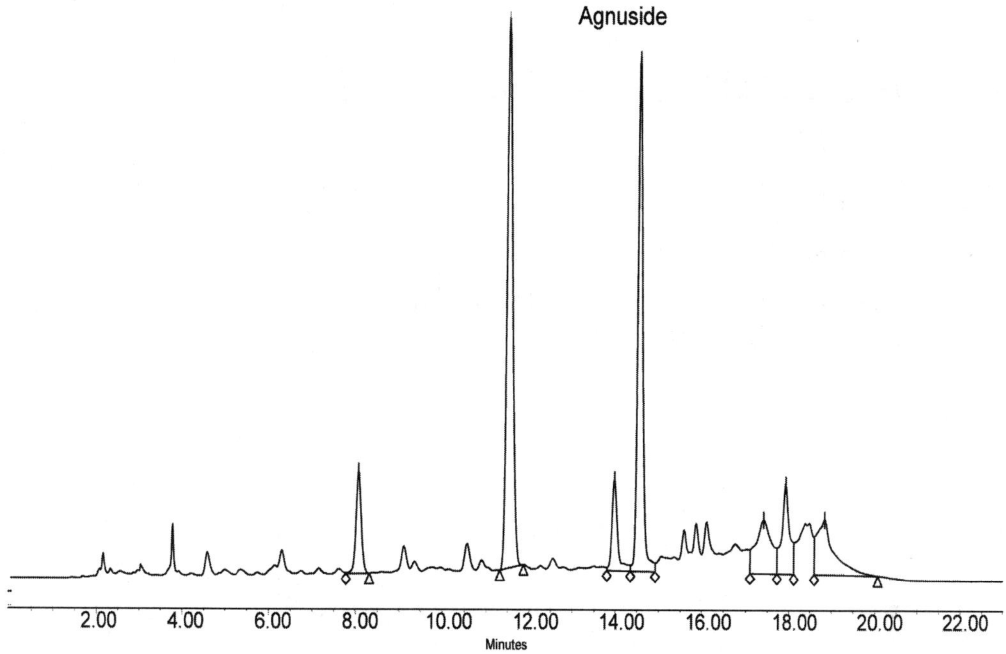

Representative HPLC chromatogram of chaste tree berries run by method 4.

References

1. Wuttke W, Jarry H, Christoffel V, et al. Chaste tree (*Vitex agnus-castus*)—pharmacology and clinical indications. *Phytomedicine*. 2003;10(4):348–57.
2. Lauritzen C, Reuter HD, Repges R, et al. Treatment of premenstrual tension syndrome with *Vitex agnus-castus*. Controlled, double-blind study versus pyridoxine. *Phytomedicine*. 1997;4(3):183–9.
3. Loch EG, Selle H, Boblitz N. Treatment of premenstrual syndrome with a phytopharmaceutical formulation containing *Vitex agnus-castus*. *J Women Health Gend-Based Med*. 2000;9(3):315–20.
4. Hoberg E, Orjala J, Meier B, et al. Diterpenoids from the fruits of *Vitex agnus-castus*. *Phytochemistry*. 1999;52(8):1555–8.
5. Hoberg E, Orjala J, Meier B, et al. Corrigendum to "Diterpenoids from the fruits of *Vitex agnus-castus*." *Phytochemistry*. 1999;52:1555–8. *Phytochemistry*. 2003,63(3):375.
6. Li SH, Zhang HJ, Qiu SX, et al. Vitexlactam A, a novel labdane diterpene lactam from the fruits of *Vitex agnus-castus*. *Tetrahedron Lett*. 2002;43(29):5131–4.
7. Hirobe C, Qiao ZS, Takeya K, et al. Cytotoxic flavonoids from *Vitex agnus-castus*. *Phytochemistry*. 1997;46(3):521–4.
8. Kuruuzum-Uz A, Stroch K, Demirezer LO, et al. Glucosides from *Vitex agnus-castus*. *Phytochemistry*. 2003;63(8):959–64.
9. Sorensen JM, Katsiotis ST. Variation in essential oil yield and composition of Cretan *Vitex agnus-castus* L. fruits. *J Essential Oil Res*. 1999;11(5):599–605.
10. Hoberg E, Meier B, Sticher O, et al. Quantitative high-performance liquid chromatographic analysis of casticin in the fruits of *Vitex agnus-castus*. *Pharm Biol* (Lisse, Netherlands). 2001;39(1):57–61.
11. Hoberg E, Meier B, Sticher O. Quantitative high-performance liquid chromatographic analysis of diterpenoids in *agni-casti fructus*. *Planta Med*. 2000;66(4):352–5.

CHONDROITIN SULFATE

Description

Common name: Chondroitinsulfuric acid

Molecular weight: Varies, depending upon source and method of extraction/purification, up to 50,000.

Chemical formula: Chondroitin sulfate is a polymeric sulfated glycosaminoglycan.

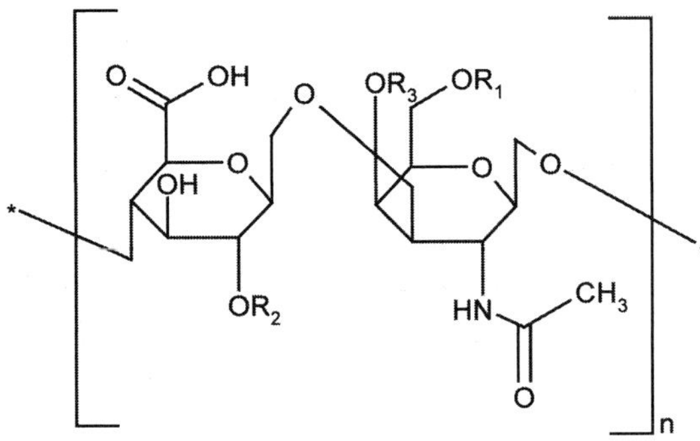

R_1, R_2, and R_3 can be either H or SO_3
Chondroitin sulfate

Solubility: Very water soluble, insoluble in organic solvents.

Other physical/chemical data: No significant UV absorption above 210 nm; very hygroscopic.

Uses: Used in dietary supplements to help relieve symptoms of osteoarthritis. It is often found in dietary supplements in conjunction with glucosamine.

Mode of Action

Chondroitin sulfate supplements may relieve symptoms of osteoarthritis by increasing levels of chondroitin sulfate in articular cartilage and may inhibit enzymes that are responsible for cartilage deterioration. Chondroitin sulfate may also increase bioavailability of glucosamine.

Methods of Analysis

Chondroitin sulfate has been difficult to analyze in dietary supplements for several reasons. It is a polymer with a wide molecular weight range and has virtually no chromaphore, and the sulfate groups make it extremely hydrophilic.

In addition, the structure of chondroitin sulfate is similar to other glycosaminoglycan polymers, such as keratan sulfate, heparin, and heparin sulfate, which may be present as impurities or adulterants. Four general techniques have been used to characterize and quantify chondroitin sulfate in dietary supplements: carbazole reaction, cetyl pyridinium chloride (CPC) titration, size-exclusion chromatography, and enzymatic hydrolysis followed by HPLC.

Carbazole reaction: In the carbazole titration method,[1] chondroitin sulfate is treated with sulfuric acid and heated to hydrolyze the chondroitin sulfate to hexuronic acid and hexosamine. Carbazole is then added and reacts with the hexuronic acid to form a colored product that can be measured by colorimetry. Although relatively easy to use and rugged, the method is nonspecific; any other compounds containing hexuronic acid moieties, such as glycosaminoglycans, will react with the carbazole to give a positive response.

Standard and sample preparation: Add about 0.5 mL of standard or sample solution containing about 0.05 to 0.5 mg/mL of chondroitin sulfate to a test tube containing about 5.5 mL of sulfuric acid–water (6:1) that is immersed in an ice bath. Allow the solution to warm to room temperature, and then place the test tube in a water bath at 60°C for 90 seconds. Cool to room temperature, add 200 µL of a 0.1% solution of carbazole, and shake vigorously. After 1 hour, measure the absorption of the solution at 527 nm.

CPC titration: Cetyl pyridinium chloride (CPC) is a positively charged polymer that will form an ion-pair with chondroitin sulfate. This ion-pair is insoluble in water and will cause turbidity. By titrating a solution of chondroitin sulfate and measuring the resulting turbidity with a phototrode, the amount of chondroitin sulfate can be determined. The technique[2] is reproducible, but it has several drawbacks. Like the carbazole reaction technique, it is subject to interferences from other glycosaminoglycans, as well as other large, anionic molecules, such as surfactants and some proteins. Very low molecular weight chondroitin sulfate may not yield a positive response. Lastly, the CPC titrant requires special safety precautions and disposal procedures.

Standard and sample preparation: Prepare both samples and chondroitin sulfate standard in a dilute phosphate buffer (pH 7.2) at a concentration of 1 mg/mL. Transfer 5 mL of standard or sample to a titration vessel with about 30 mL of water. Titrate the solution with a 1-mg/mL solution of cetylpyridinium chloride in water. The end point can be determined visually, or, if using an automatic titrator with a phototrode detector in transmittance mode, the end point can be determined automatically.

Size-exclusion chromatography: Because chondroitin sulfate is a polymeric species, size-exclusion chromatography (SEC) can be used to separate it from small molecules often found in dietary supplements. Its lack of a chromaphore, however, necessitates use of either short-wavelength UV detection (<210 nm) or refractive index detection. In addition, SEC cannot distinguish between chondroitin sulfate and other polymers of similar size; therefore, its selectivity is not very good.

Way et al.[3] presented a method using SEC for the assay of chondroitin sulfate in dietary supplements. They noted, however, that the presence of other glycosaminoglycans in the samples could cause overestimation of the chondroitin sulfate content.

Standard and sample preparation: Dissolve standards and samples in water. Prepare linearity standard concentrations ranging from 0.2 to 0.8 mg/mL. Prepare samples so that the final chondroitin sulfate concentration is about 0.4 mg/mL.

Chromatography

Column: Phenomenex BioSep-SEC-S2000, 300 × 7.8 mm.

Mobile phase: 0.1 M sodium phosphate, pH 7.0.

Flow rate: 0.8 mL/minute

Injection: 50 µL

Detection wavelength: UV at 207 nm

Validation data:

Linearity: Correlation coefficient >0.999.

Accuracy: 98.7% average recovery of spiked samples.

Precision: 2.48% RSD for 10 samples.

Selectivity: It was demonstrated that ingredients magnesium stearate, manganese ascorbate, and glucosamine hydrochloride did not interfere.

Ruggedness: 104.8% of first analysis

Robustness: Not specified

LOD/LOQ: Not specified

Enzymatic hydrolysis with HPLC: Chondroitin sulfate can be hydrolyzed to disaccharide units by the enzyme chondroitinase ABC.[4] The resulting disaccharide units are unsaturated, with a UV absorbance maximum of 232 nm:

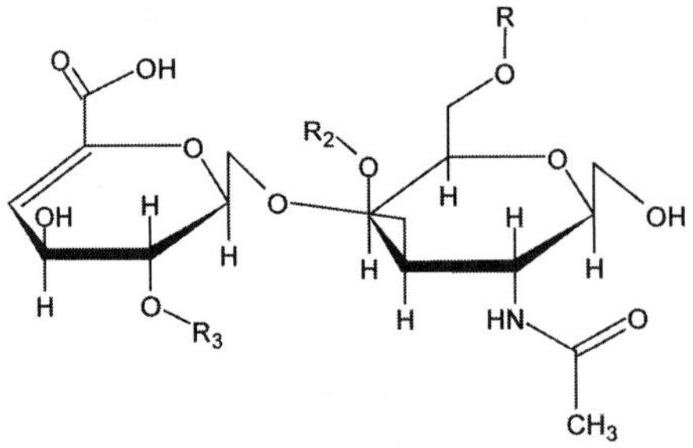

	R	R_2	R_3
Di-0S	H	H	H
Di-4S	H	SO_3	H
Di-6S	SO_3	H	H

Enzymatic hydrolysis using chondroitinase ABC followed by HPLC offers several advantages compared to other techniques for characterizing chondroitin sulfate. Chondroitinase ABC will only hydrolyze chondroitin sulfate, allowing the method to distinguish between chondroitin sulfate and related glycosaminoglycans. In addition, the ratios of the resulting disaccharide units can be used to determine the source of the chondroitin sulfate (e.g., bovine, porcine, avian, or shark).[5,6] The disaccharides can be separated by ion-exchange, ion-pair, or normal-phase HPLC, with detection at 232 nm, allowing for easy quantitation. Ion-exchange chromatography using amino columns has been most widely used for the separation of the disaccharides. The major disadvantage to the technique is the cost and availability of the chondroitinase ABC enzyme. Typical ion-exchange chromatographic conditions for the separation of the disaccharides are given.

Chromatography

Column: Phenosphere NH_2, 5 μm, 150 × 4.6 mm.

Mobile phase: Acetonitrile–0.08 M sodium acetate buffer (pH 5.0) (30:70).

Flow rate: 1.5 mL/minute

Injection volume: 30 μL

Detection wavelength: 240 nm

Run time: 20 minutes

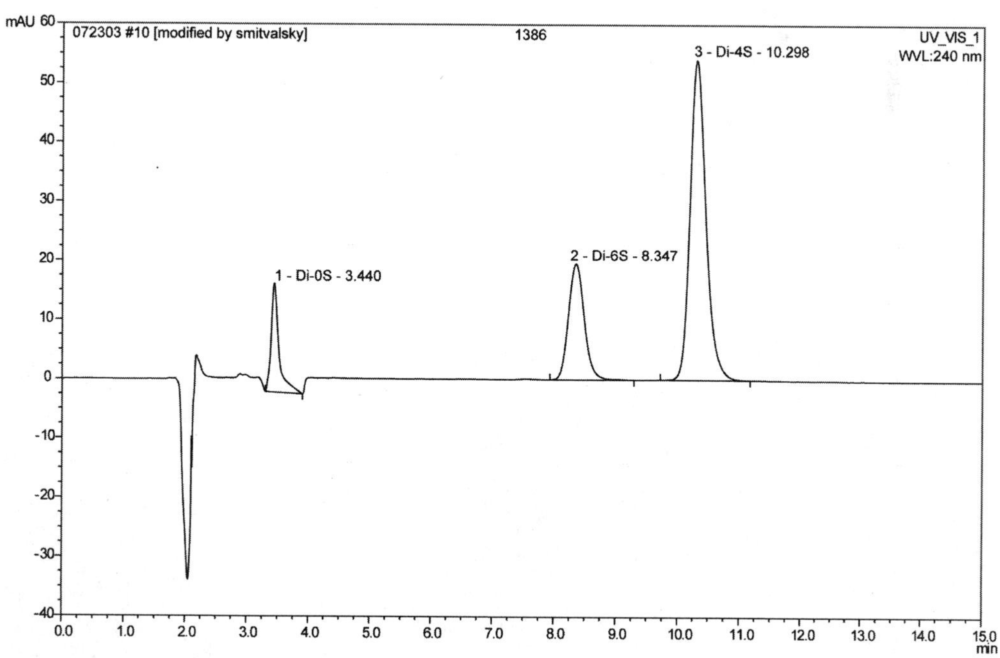

Typical HPLC chromatogram of chondroitin sulfate using enzymatic hydrolysis method.

References

1. Dische Z. A modificatation of the carbazole reaction of hexuronic acids for the study of polyuronides. *J Biol Chem.* 1950;183:489–94.
2. Institute for Nutraceutical Advancement method 120.002, www.nsf.org/business/ina/index.asp?program=INA.
3. Way WK, Gibson KG, Breite A. Determination of chondroitin sulfate in nutritional supplements by liquid chromatography. *J Liq Chromatogr Relat Technol.* 2000;23(18):2851–60.
4. Ototani N, Sato N, Yosizawa Z. High-performance liquid chromatography of unsaturated disaccharides produced from chondroitin sulfate by chondroitinase. *J Biochem.* 1979;85:1383–5.
5. Karamanos NK, Syrokou A, Vanky P, et al. Determination of 24 variously sulfated galactosaminoglycan- and hyaluronan-derived disaccharides by high-performance liquid chromatography. *Anal Biochem.* 1994;221:189–99.
6. Volpi N. Hyaluronic acid and chondroitin sulfate–unsaturated disaccharides analysis by high-performance liquid chromatography and fluorometric determination with dansylhydrazine. *Anal Biochem.* 2000;277:19–24.

COENZYME Q_{10}

Description

Chemical name: 2-(3,7,11,15,19,23,27,31,35,39-decamethyl-2,6,10,14,18,22,26,30,34,38-tetracontadecaenyl)-5,6-dimethoxy-3-methylbenzo-1,4-quinone

Common names: Coenzyme Q-199, CoQ10, ubidecarenone, ubiquinone 50

Molecular weight: 863.34

Chemical formula: $C_{59}H_{90}O_4$

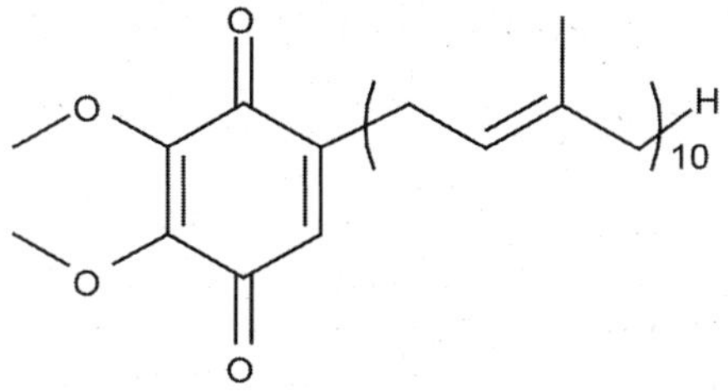

Coenzyme Q_{10}

Solubility: Soluble in ethanol, isopropanol, chloroform, hexane, and other organic solvents.

Other physical/chemical data: UV max = 272 nm (ε = 14,400), 325 nm (ε = 1340); melting point = 49°C to 50°C.

Uses: Coenzyme Q_{10} (CoQ10) is a naturally occurring antioxidant. As a dietary supplement, it is used to prevent or to treat congestive heart failure, to delay the onset of Parkinson's syndrome, and to prevent or to treat certain forms of cancer.

Mode of Action

CoQ10 is a powerful antioxidant that acts as an electron shuttle between flavoproteins and cytochromes in the electron-transport chain. It is the only electron shuttle that is not covalently bonded or tightly bound to a protein. CoQ10 is critical in the oxidation–reduction of FeS in iron–sulfur proteins.

Methods of Analysis

A few methods have been published for the analysis of CoQ10 in dietary supplements; many more have been published for the analysis of CoQ10 in biological samples. Both reversed-phase and normal-phase HPLC with UV detection can be used to quantify CoQ10 in dietary supplements.

CoQ10 is both oxygen- and light-sensitive; therefore, low-actinic glassware and degassed solvents should be used throughout the analysis.

Method: Andersson[1] used nonaqueous reversed-phase HPLC to separate CoQ10 from degradation products in raw materials, soy bean oil formulations, and micelle-based preparations. It was found that the nonaqueous reversed-phase system provided better retention time stability and selectivity than normal-phase systems. The method was able to separate CoQ10 (oxidized) from CoQ10 (reduced), coenzyme Q9 (oxidized), coenzyme Q9 (reduced), and ubichromenol.

Sample preparation: Prepare soy bean oil capsules containing CoQ10 by transferring the fill material into a 100-mL volumetric flask with 20 mL of hexane, sonicating, and diluting to volume with methanol. Dilute a 2-mL aliquot to 50 mL with methanol and inject into the HPLC system.

For micelle-based preparations, dissolve a 100-mg sample in 100 mL of 20% n-hexane in methanol and sonicate for 5 minutes. Inject this solution.

Chromatography

Column: Spherisorb ODS-2, 3 µm, 100 × 4.6 mm.

Mobile phase: 10% n-hexane in methanol

Flow rate: 1.4 mL/minute

Column temperature: Not available

Injection volume: 20 µL

Detection wavelength: 275 nm

Validation data:

Linearity: 0.2 to 100 mcg/mL

Accuracy: 100.3±1.9% (n = 6) recovery of CoQ10 from spiked placebo capsules, 99.7±2.5% (n = 8) recovery of CoQ10 from spiked micelle vehicle.

Precision: 2% RSD (n = 11) for soy bean capsules, 2.6% RSD (n = 6) for micelle-based preparations.

Selectivity: Light stressing followed by HPLC with diode-array detection was used to show separation of CoQ10 from degradation products and related compounds.

Ruggedness: Not determined

Robustness: Not determined

LOD/LOQ: LOD = 2 ng

Reference

1. Andersson S. Determination of coenzyme Q by non-aqueous reversed-phase liquid chromatography. *J Chromatogr A*. 1992;606:272–6.

DEVIL'S CLAW

Description

Botanical name: *Harpagophytum procumbens*

Common name: Devil's Claw

Parts of plant used: Tubers and roots

Uses: As an anti-inflammatory agent to treat arthritis and rheumatism and to alleviate back pain.

Mode of Action

Several clinical trials have proven that devil's claw root extracts are effective in fighting osteoarthritis, alleviating back pain, and treating low back pain.[1–5] Although the mechanism of devil's claw's anti-inflammatory activity is still unclear, extracts of devil's claw were found to inhibit TNF-α synthesis in LPS-stimulated primary human monocytes.[6] The major iridoid harpagoside has not been proven clinically to be the active component in devil's claw, but generally iridoids are believed to contribute to the total anti-inflammatory effect.

Chemical Markers

Iridoids are believed to be the major chemical components in devil's claw with harpagoside as the dominant iridoid. Other iridoids purified from devil's claw include procumbide and its 6′-O-p-coumaroyl ester, procumboside, 8-O-(p-coumaroyl)-harpagide.[7–9] Several phenylpropanic acid glycosides (aceteoside, isoacetoside, verbascoside, 6-acetylacteoside, 2,6-diacetylacteoside) were also identified from the root extract.[7–10] Other compounds include sterols, triterpenes, phenolic acid, flavonoids, and a phenylethanoic derivative.[8,11,12] In the U.S. market, harpagoside is used as marker compound for quality control of devil's claw.

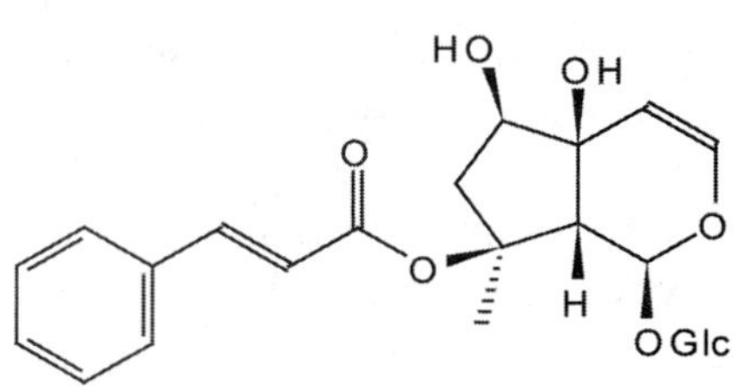

Harpagoside

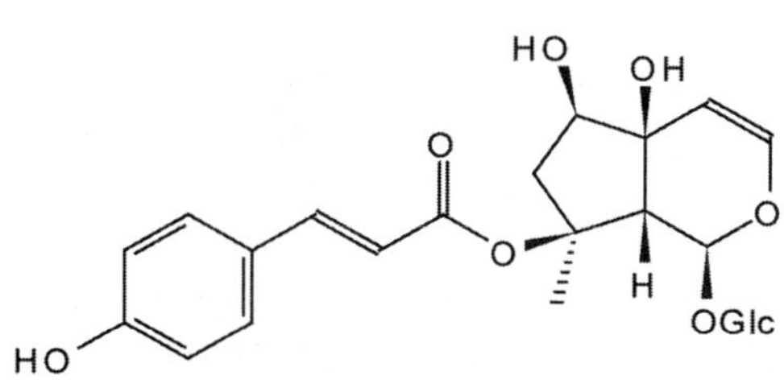

8-O-(p-Coumaroyl)-harpagide

Methods of Analysis

Various methods have been used to analyze the iridoids in the root of devil's claw including HPLC with UV detection, HPTLC methods with UV detection and visualization with sulfuric acid, a colorimetric method to determine the total glucoiridoids, and GC to analyze the silyl derivatives.[13–19] HPLC is the most accepted method. Various solvents have been used to extract iridoids from the root of devil's claw including hot water, methanol, and aqueous alcohol solutions.

Method 1: The method of Baghdikian et al.[15] was used. This method analyzes two iridoids, harpagoside and 8-O-(p-coumaroyl)-harpagide in two species Harpagophytum procumbens and Harpagophytum zeyheri.

Sample preparation: Infuse powdered roots in boiling water (500 mL) and then macerate for 12 hours at 40°C.

Chromatography

Column: Waters µBondapak C18 10 µm, 300 × 3.9 mm with a precolumn Guard Pak µBondapak C18.

Mobile phase: Water–methanol (43:57) isocratic.

Flow rate: 1.0 mL/minute

Injection volume: 20 µL

Detection wavelength: 278 nm

Validation data:

Linearity: Not specified

Accuracy: Not specified

Precision: RSD 2.92% for harpagoside and RSD 1.46% for 8-O-(p-coumaroyl)-harpagide.

Selectivity: Peak identification was determined against standards.

Ruggedness: Not specified

Robustness: Not specified

LOD/LOQ: Not specified

Method 2: The method of Guillerault et al.[17] was used. This method analyzes three iridoids, harpagoside, harpagide, and 8-O-(p-coumaroyl)-harpagide, with two detection methods: UV and light scattering.

Sample preparation: For drugs, add 5 g of drug to 70 mL of methanol, warm for 15 minutes, filter, and then evaporate in vacuo. Dissolve the residue in 50 mL of water, and concentrate 2 mL of this preparation on SEP PACK. Elute with 10 mL of water and methanol separately. Evaporate the methanol part under vacuum and dissolve in 0.5 mL of water for HPLC.

For the extract, disperse 5 g in 100 mL of water, and concentrate 2 mL of the extraction solution and prepare as for drugs.

Chromatography

Column: Phenomenex Bondclone, C18, 10 µm, 300 × 3.9 mm.

Mobile phase: Water–methanol

Gradient: 0 to 10 minutes, 15% methanol; 10 to 45 minutes, 50% methanol; and 45 to 60 minutes, 15% methanol.

Flow rate: 1.0 mL/minute

Injection volume: 20 µL

Detection wavelength: 270, 305, and 312 nm for harpagoside and 8-O-(p-coumaroyl)-harpagide and light scattering for harpagide.

Validation data:

Linearity: 0.041 to 0.5 mg/mL for 8-O-(p-coumaroyl)-harpagide and 0.1 to 0.8 mg/mL for harpagide, and 0.13 to 1 mg/mL for harpagoside by light-scattering detection.

Accuracy: Not specified

Precision: RSD all less than 5% for the different detection methods.

Selectivity: Peak identification was determined against standards.

Ruggedness: Not specified

Robustness: Not specified

LOD/LOQ: Limit of detection for 8-O-(p-coumaroyl)-harpagide was 2 mcg/mL by UV at 312 and 50 mcg/mL by light scattering; for harpagoside it was 4 mcg/mL by UV at 278 nm and 50 mcg/mL by light scattering; and for harpagide it was 60 mcg/mL by light-scattering detection.

Method 3: The unpublished method of Mingfu Wang was used.

Sample preparation: Weigh 300-mg samples, add 35 mL of methanol, sonicate for 25 minutes, and shake for 15 minutes. Allow the flask to cool to room temperature, and fill to volume (50 mL) with methanol.

Chromatography

Column: Phenomenex Luna C18 (2), 5 µm, 250 × 4.6 mm.

Mobile phase: Water (adjusted to pH 2.5 with phosphoric acid)–methanol isocratic (34:66).

Flow rate: 0.8 mL/minute

Injection volume: 10 µL

Detection wavelength: 278 nm

Validation data: Not available

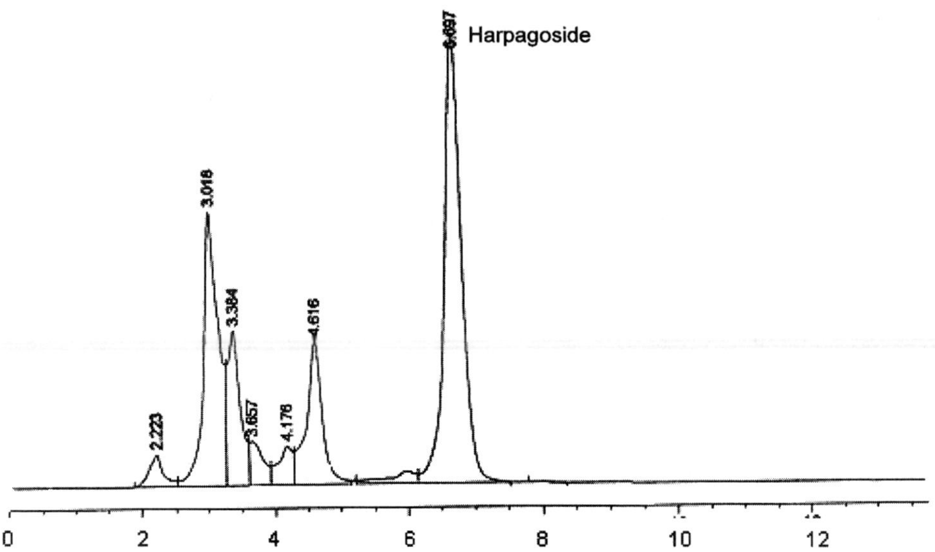

Representative HPLC chromatogram of devil's claw run by method 3.

References

1. Chrubasik S, Conradt C, Black A. The quality of clinical trials with *Harpagophytum procumbens*. *Phytomedicine*. 2003;10(6–7):613–23.
2. Chrubasik S, Model A, Black A, et al. A randomized double-blind pilot study comparing Doloteffin and Vioxx in the treatment of low back pain. *Rheumatology* (Oxford, United Kingdom). 2003;42(1):141–8.
3. Chrubasik S, Thanner J, Kunzel O, et al. Comparison of outcome measures during treatment with the proprietary *Harpagophytum* extract Doloteffin in patients with pain in the lower back, knee, or hip. *Phytomedicine*. 2002;9(3):181–94.
4. Laudahn D, Walper A. Efficacy and tolerance of *Harpagophytum* extract LI 174 in patients with chronic non-radicular back pain. *Phytother Res*. 2001;15(7):621–4.
5. Grahame R, Robinson BV. Devil's claw (*Harpagophytum procumbens*): pharmacological and clinical studies. *Ann Rheum Dis*. 1981;40(6):632.
6. Fiebich BL, Heinrich M, Hiller KO, et al. Inhibition of TNF-α synthesis in LPS-stimulated primary human monocytes by *Harpagophytum* extract SteiHap 69. *Phytomedicine*. 2001;8(1):28–30.
7. Munkombwe NM. Acetylated phenolic glycosides from *Harpagophytum procumbens*. *Phytochemistry*. 2003;62(8):1231–4.
8. Burger JF, Brandt EV, Ferreira D. Iridoid and phenolic glycosides from *Harpagophytum procumbens*. *Phytochemistry*. 1987;26(5):1453–7.
9. Kikuchi T, Matsuda S, Kubo Y, et al. New iridoid glucosides from *Harpagophytum procumbens* DC. *Chem Pharm Bull*. 1983;31(7):2296–301.
10. Ziller KH, Franz G. Analysis of the water soluble fraction from the roots of *Harpagophytum procumbens*. *Planta Med*. 1979;37(4):340–8.
11. Tunmann P, Bauersfeld HJ. Constituents of the roots of *Harpagophytum procumbens*. *Arch Pharm*. 1975;308(8):655–7.
12. Bruneton J. *Pharmacognosy, Phytochemistry, Medicinal Plants*. Paris: Lavoisier Publishing; 1995:485–7.
13. Qian H, Xie P. TLC analysis of harpagoside in devil's claw extract and its tablets. *China Journal of Chinese Materia Medica*. 1998;23(12):726–9, 764.

14. Eich J, Schmidt M, Betti G. HPLC analysis of iridoid compounds of *Harpagophytum* taxa. Quality control of pharmaceutical drug material. *Pharm Pharmacol Lett.* 1998;8(2):75–8.
15. Baghdikian B, Lanhers MC, Fleurentin J, et al. An analytical study, anti-inflammatory and analgesic effects of *Harpagophytum procumbens* and *H. zeyheri*. *Planta Med.* 1997;63(2):171–6.
16. Poukens-Renwart P, Tits M, Angenot L. Quantitative densitometric evaluation of harpagoside in the secondary roots of *Harpagophytum procumbens* DC. *J Planar Chromat.* 1996;9(3):199–202.
17. Guillerault L, Ollivier E, Elias R, et al. Determination of harpagide, 8-para-coumaroyl harpagide, and harpagoside by high-performance liquid chromatography in *Harpagophytum procumbens* drugs and in a commercial extract. *J Liq Chromatogr.* 1994;17(13): 2951–60.
18. Vanhaelen M, Vanhaelen-Fastre R, Elchami AA. Gas-liquid chromatographic determination of the iridoid content in *Harpagophytum procumbens* DC. *J Chromatogr A.* 1981;209(3):476–8.
19. Haag-Berrurier M, Kuballa B, Anton R. Determination of total glucoiridoids in the roots of *Harpagophytum procumbens* DC. *Plantes Med Phytother.* 1978;12(3):197–206.

ECHINACEA

Description

Botanical names: *Echinacea* spp.; *Echinacea purpurea; Echinacea pallida; Echinacea angustifolia.*

Common names: Narrow-leaf echinacea and narrow-leaf purple echinacea for *Echinacea angustifolia*; pale purple coneflower for *Echinacea pallida*; purple coneflower for *Echinacea purpurea*

Parts of plant used: Aerial parts and roots

Uses: As an immunostimulating agent; treatment of infections of the upper respiratory tract.

Mode of Action

More than 20 clinical trials have been performed on echinacea; most of them found positive effects for symptoms related to colds, upper respiratory tract infections, and flu. There is the widespread belief that echinacea has immunomodulatory activity; however, it is still somewhat unclear which compounds are responsible for this activity. Polysaccharides, alkamides, or the caffeic acid derivatives may be active components.[1]

Chemical Markers

Various chemical compounds have been identified from *Echinacea* spp. including alkamides, polyalkenes, polyalkynes, volatile oils, phenolic compounds, and polysaccharides. More than 20 alkamides have been identified in *Echinacea* spp. Most of them are isobutylamides of C11–C16 long-chain unsaturated fatty acids, with a mixture of isomeric dodeca-2,4,8,10-tetraenoic acid isobutylamides as the major ones. The root contains higher amounts of alkamides than other parts and the highest concentration is found in *Echinacea angustifolia*. Echinacea is also known to contain phenolic compounds (flavonoids and caffeic acid derivatives). The well-known caffeic acid derivatives found in echinacea are cichoric acid, echinacoside, 1,3-dicaffeoylquinic acid, and chlorogenic acid; caftaric acid with cichoric acid as the major phenolic compound in *Echinacea purpurea* and echinacoside as the main phenolic compound in *E. angustifolia* and *E. pallida*.[2] Currently, the alkamides and caffeic acid derivatives are used as marker compounds for quality control of echinacea products.

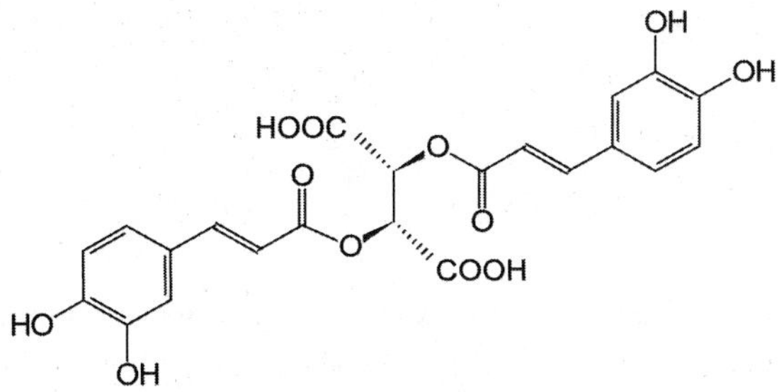

Cichoric acid

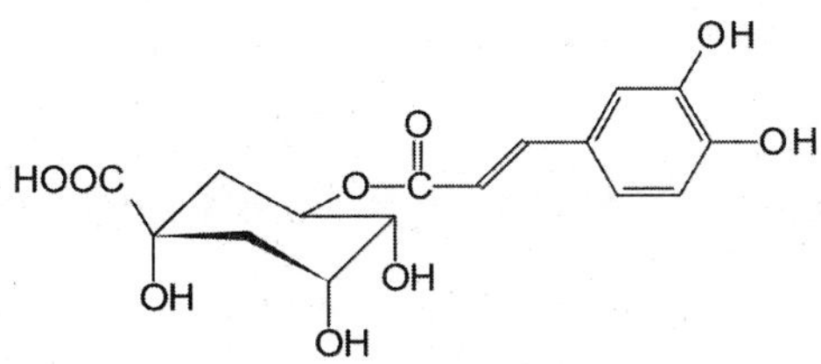

Chlorogenic acid

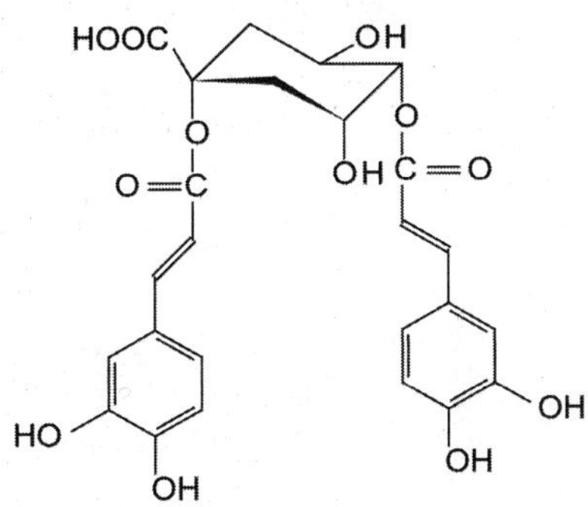

1,3-Dicaffeoylquinic acid

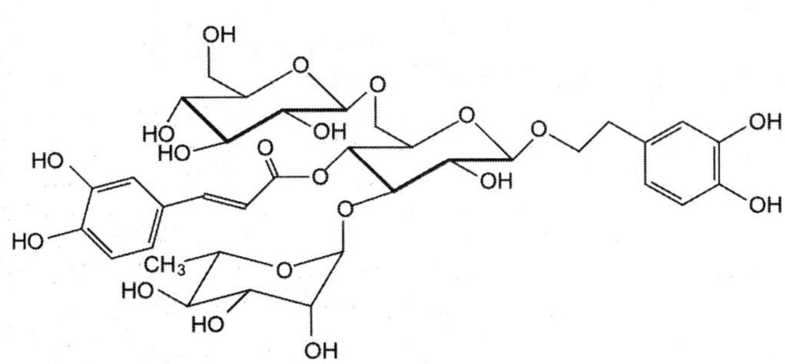

Echinacoside

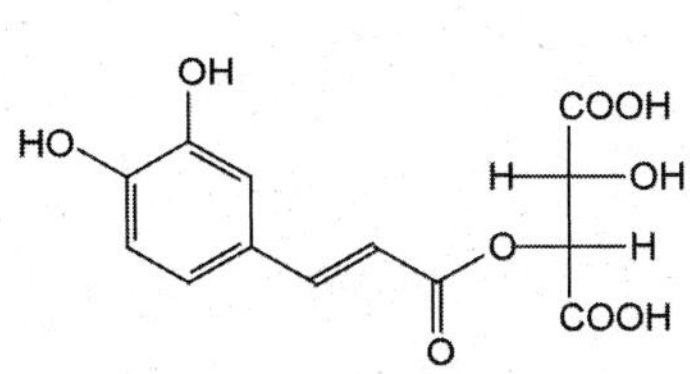

Caftaric acid

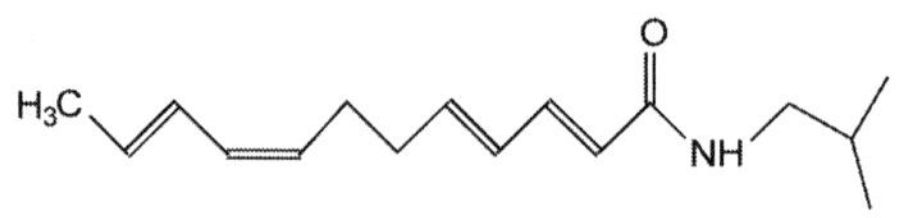

Dodeca-2E,4E,8Z,10E-tetraenoic acid isobutylamide

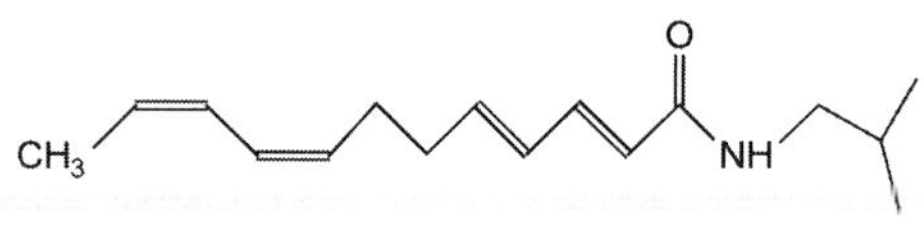

Dodeca-2E,4E,8Z,10Z-tetraenoic acid isobutylamide

Methods of Analysis

As echinacea is one of the most popular herbs in the U.S. and European markets, various analytical techniques including TLC, HPLC, micellar electrokinetic chromatography, and ATR–IR and NIR spectroscopy have been used to analyze the compounds in echinacea.[3–6] Currently, HPLC is the most accepted method for analysis of alkamides and caffeic acid derivatives in *Echinacea* spp.

Method 1: The method found at www.nsfina.org determines 2-O-caffeoyltartaric acid (caftaric acid), 2,3-O-dicaffeoyltartartic acid (cichoric acid or chicoric acid), 3-O-caffeoylquinic acid (chlorogenic acid), and echinacoside in plant materials and powdered extracts of *Echinacea angustifolia, E. pallida,* and *E. purpurea.*

Sample preparation: For plant material, shake 0.125 g of ground material with 25 mL of ethanol–water (70:30) for 15 minutes.

For extracts, shake 0.06 g of extract with 25 mL of ethanol–water (70:30) for 15 minutes.

Chromatography

Column: Phenomenex Prodigy ODS(3), 5 μm, 100Å, 250 × 4.6 mm.

Mobile phase: Solvent A = water (0.1% phosphoric acid), solvent B = acetonitrile.

Gradient:

Time (minutes)	%A	%B
0	90	10
13	78	22
14	60	40
14.5	60	40
15	90	10

Injection volume: 5 µL
Run time: 20 minutes
Flow rate: 1.5 mL/minute
Column temperature: 35°C
Detection wavelength: 330 nm

Validation data: Not available, but this method is known to be a fully validated method.

Method 2: The method of Molgaard et al.[7] can be used to analyze cichoric acid, 1,3-dicaffeoylquinic acid, echinacoside, and alkamides in *Echinacea purpurea* simultaneously.

Sample preparation: For plant material and capsules, sonicate about 400 mg of sample in 10 mL of methanol–water (7:3) for 30 minutes, and follow by 120 minutes on a blood turner.

For liquid samples, dilute the samples with extraction solvent.

Chromatography

Column: Merck LiChroCART Superspher 100 RP-18 column, 5 µm, 125 × 4.1 mm.

Mobile phase: Solvent A = water–acetonitrile (95:5), solvent B = water–acetonitrile (5:95), solvent C = water–acetonitrile (95:5) with 0.1% trifluoroacetic acid.

Gradient:

Time (minutes)	%A	%B	%C
0	75	5	20
4	75	5	20
4		curve-2*	
7	68	12	20
19	60	20	20
19		curve-2*	
30	49	31	20
30		curve-2*	
55	27	53	20

* Convex/concave curves as described in Shimadzu's Class-LC-10 software.

Flow rate: 1.3 mL/minute
Injection volume: 5 µL
Column temperature: 40°C
Detection wavelength: 0 to 35 minutes = 290 nm, 35 to 55 minutes = 260 nm.

Validation data:

Linearity: Not available

Accuracy: The percent recoveries were 95 for cichoric acid, 98 for dodeca-2E,4E-8Z,10E/Z-tetraenisobutylamide, and more than 80 for undeca-2Z,4E-dien-8,10-diynisobutylamide.

Precision: The RSD was less than 2% for all four compounds.

Selectivity: Peak identification was determined against standards.

Ruggedness: The RSD was less than 1%.

Robustness: The RSD was less than 5%.

LOD/LOQ: LOD for cichoric acid, dodeca-2E,4E-8Z,10E/Z-tetraenisobutylamide, and undeca-2Z,4E-dien-8,10-diynisobutylamide were 0.011, 0.000074, and 0.0011 mg/mL, respectively. The LOQs were 0.038, 0.000025, and 0.0037, respectively.

Method 3: The method of Laasonen et al.[3,4] can be used for the simultaneous analysis of alkamides and caffeic acid derivatives in *Echinacea purpurea, E. angustifolia, E. pallida,* and *Parthenium integrifolium.*

Sample preparation: Extract 100 mg of herbal powder with 8 mL of ethanol–water (70:30) three times by sonication for 5 minutes and then centrifuge. Combine the supernates and adjust to a volume of 25 mL.

Chromatography

Column: Phenomenex Luna C18, 3 μm, 100 × 4.6 mm.

Mobile phase: Solvent A = water (0.1% phosphoric acid), solvent B = acetonitrile.

Gradient:

Time (minutes)	%A	%B
0	95	5
2	82	18
4	82	18
7	30	70
20	10	90

Flow rate: 1.0 mL/minute

Injection volume: 25 μL

Detection wavelength: 255 nm

Validation data: Not available

Method 4: The method of Luo et al.[8] also can be used to analyze alkamides and caffeic acid derivatives in *Echinacea purpurea* simultaneously.

Sample preparation: Sonicate 1 g of ground plant materials in 10 mL of methanol– water (0.1% phosphoric acid) (70:30) for 20 minutes.

Chromatography

Column: Johnson Spherigel C18, 5 μm, 250 × 4.6 mm.

Mobile phase: Solvent A = water (0.1% formic acid), solvent B = acetonitrile.

Gradient:

Time (minutes)	%A	%B
0	90	10
9	81.5	18.5
9.5	55	45
39.5	20	80
42	0	100
45	90	10

Flow rate: 1 mL/minute

Injection volume: 10 μL

Detection wavelength: 330 nm for caffeic acid derivatives and 254 nm for alkamides.

Column temperature: 30°C

Validation data:

Linearity: 600 to 1200 ng at 330 nm for cichoric acid, 300 to 900 ng at 254 nm for dodeca-2E,4E,8Z,10E-tetraenoic acid isobutylamide and dodeca-2E,4E,8Z,10Z-tetraenoic acid isobutylamide.

Accuracy: The percent recoveries were 98.7 for cichoric acid and 95.7 for dodeca-2E,4E-8Z,10E/Z-tetraenisobutylamide.

Precision: Not specified

Selectivity: Peak identification was determined against standards.

Ruggedness: Not available

Robustness: Not available

LOD/LOQ: LODs for cichoric acid and dodeca-2E,4E-8Z,10E/Z-tetraenisobutylamide were 40 and 35 ng, respectively.

Method 5: The unpublished method of Mingfu Wang was used to determine the phenolic compounds in echinacea.

Sample preparation: Accurately weigh approximately 0.25 g of ground raw material or 100 mg of dried extract and place into a 50-mL volumetric flask. Add exactly 40 mL of methanol–water (70:30) and sonicate for 30 minutes. Then dilute to volume with methanol–water (70:30).

Chromatography

Column: Phenomenex Luna Phenylhexyl, 3 μm, 150 × 4.6 mm.

Mobile phase: Solvent A = water (0.2% phosphoric acid), solvent B = acetonitrile.

Gradient:

Time (minutes)	%A	%B
0	94	6
8	84	16
20	40	60
25	40	60

Injection volume: 5 μL

Detection wavelength: 330 nm

Flow rate: 1.1 mL/minute

Validation data: Not available

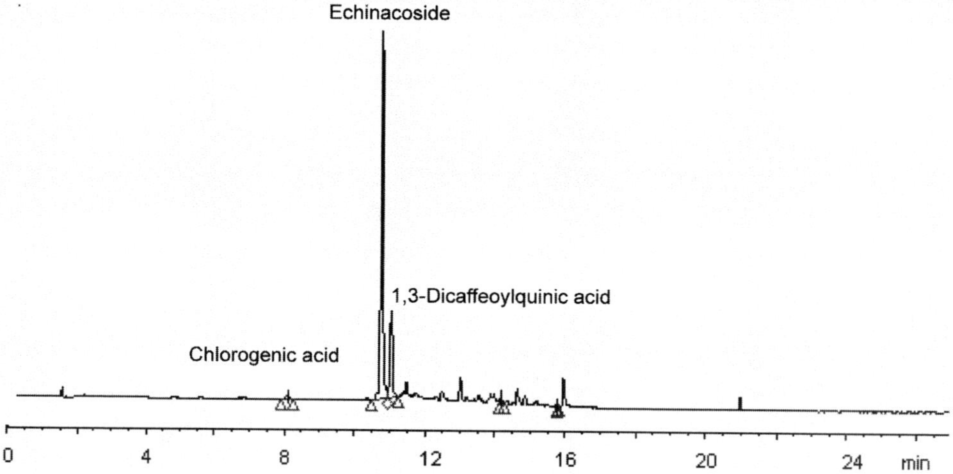

Representative HPLC chromatogram of *Echinacea angustifolia* run by method 5.

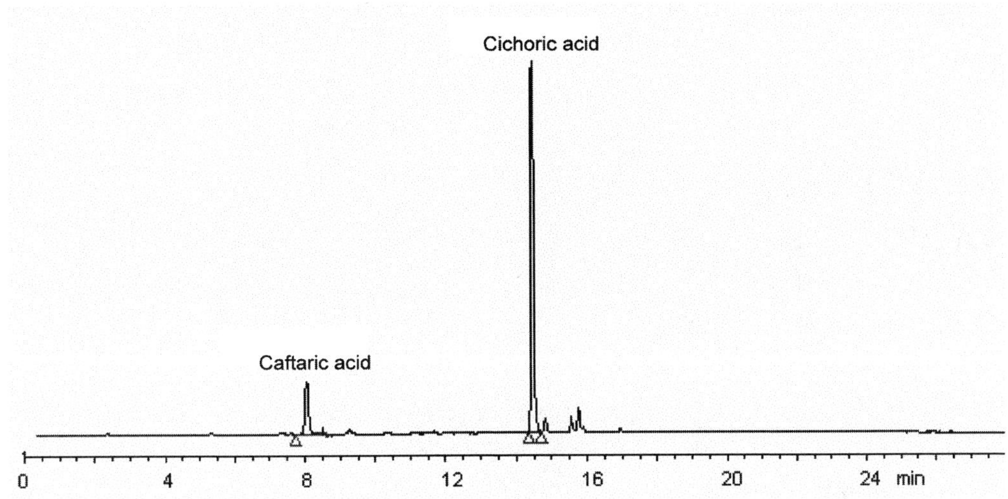

Representative HPLC chromatogram of *Echinacea purpurea* run by method 5.

References

1. Perry NB, Van Klink JW, Burgess EJ, et al. Alkamide levels in *Echinacea purpurea*. A rapid analytical method revealing differences among roots, rhizomes, stems, leaves, and flowers. *Planta Med*. 1997;63(1):58–62.
2. Perry NB, Burgess EJ, Glennie VL. Echinacea standardization: analytical methods for phenolic compounds and typical levels in medicinal species. *J Agric Food Chem*. 2001;49(4):1702–6.
3. Laasonen M, Harmia-Pulkkinen T, Simard CL, et al. Fast identification of *Echinacea purpurea* dried roots using near-infrared spectroscopy. *Anal Chem*. 2002;74(11):2493–9.
4. Laasonen M, Wennberg T, Harmia-Pulkkinen T, et al. Simultaneous analysis of alkamides and caffeic acid derivatives for the identification of *Echinacea purpurea, Echinacea angustifolia, Echinacea pallida* and *Parthenium integrifolium* roots. *Planta Med*. 2002;68(6):572–4.
5. Bergeron C, Livesey JF, Awang DV, et al. A quantitative HPLC method for the quality assurance of Echinacea products on the North American market. *Phytochem Anal*. 2000;11(4):207–15.
6. Schulz H, Pfeffer S, Quilitzsch R, et al. Rapid and non-destructive determination of the echinacoside content in Echinacea roots by ATR–IR and NIR spectroscopy. *Planta Med*. 2002;68(10):926–9.
7. Molgaard P, Johnsen S, Christensen P, et al. HPLC method validated for the simultaneous analysis of cichoric acid and alkamides in *Echinacea purpurea* plants and products. *J Agric Food Chem*. 2003;51(24):6922–33.
8. Luo XB, Chen B, Yao SZ, et al. Simultaneous analysis of caffeic acid derivatives and alkamides in roots and extracts of *Echinacea purpurea* by high-performance liquid chromatography-photodiode array detection-electrospray mass spectrometry. *J Chromatogr A*. 2003;986(1):73–81.

EPHEDRA

Description

Botanical names: *Ephedra sinica* Stapf; *Ephedra equisetina; Ephedra intermedia; Ephedra distachya*

Common name: Ma Huang

NOTE: *Ephedra nevadensis* (Mormon tea), *Ephedra antisyphilitica,* and *Ephedra trifurca* are also ephedra species; however, they do not contain the ephedrine alkaloids for which ephedra is associated and are not covered here.

Parts of plant used: Aerial parts

Uses: Treatment of asthma and bronchial spasms; as a stimulant and diaphoretic.

NOTE: In April 2004 the U.S. Food and Drug Administration prohibited the sale of dietary supplements containing ephedrine alkaloids because of concerns about their link to significant adverse health effects, including heart attack and stroke. More information is available at www.fda.gov/oc/initiatives/ephedra/february2004/finalsummary.html.

Mode of Action

Ephedrine and pseudoephedrine, two of the biogenic amines found in ephedra are potent stimulants. Ephedrine is a sympathomimetic compound that stimulates both α- and β-adrenergic receptors. Administration of ephedrine or pseudoephedrine causes cardiac stimulation, elevated systolic and diastolic blood pressure, and CNS stimulation. These biogenic amines are also believed to cause glycogenolysis and increased oxygen consumption.

Chemical Markers

Ephedra is known to contain up to six bioactive alkaloids: (–)-ephedrine, (+)-pseudoephedrine, (–)-methylephedrine, (+)-methylpseudoephedrine, (–)-norephedrine, and (+)-norpseudoephedrine. These alkaloids constitute about 1 wt% to 2.5 wt% of the plant on a dry weight basis, with (–)-ephedrine accounting for between 30% and 90% of this total. Typically, ephedrine and pseudoephedrine combined account for more than 90% of the total alkaloids in ephedra. The species *E. nevadensis, E. antisyphilitica,* and *E. trifurca,* all found in North America, have thus far been found to be free of these alkaloids.

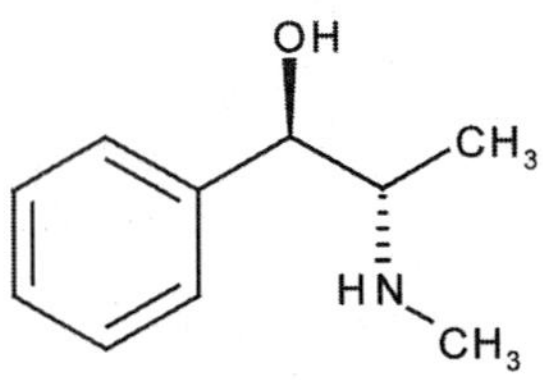

Ephedrine

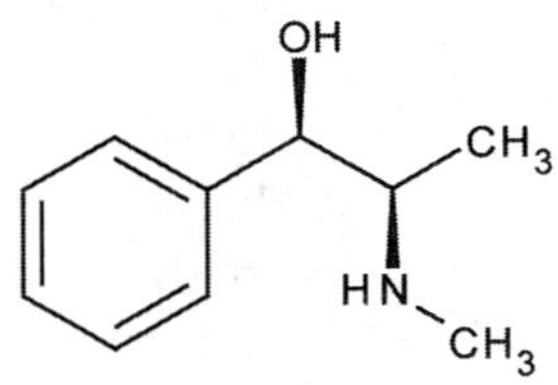

Pseudoephedrine

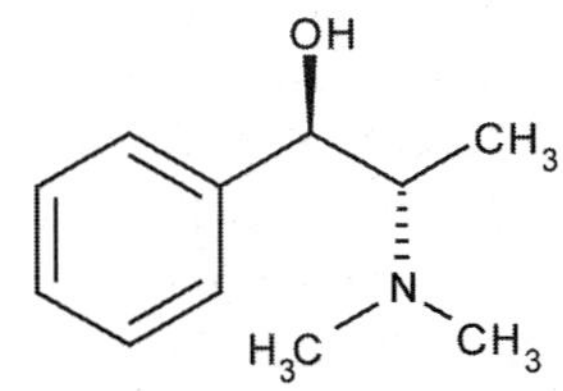

Methylephedrine

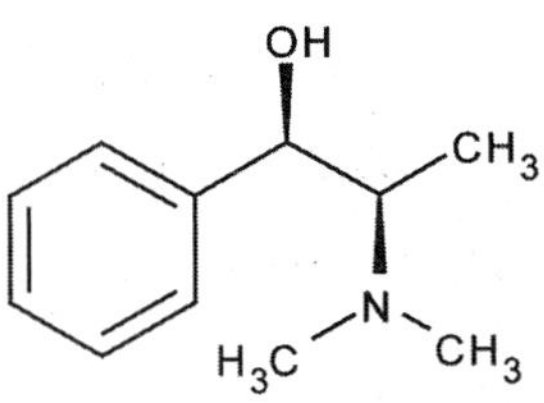

Methylpseudoephedrine

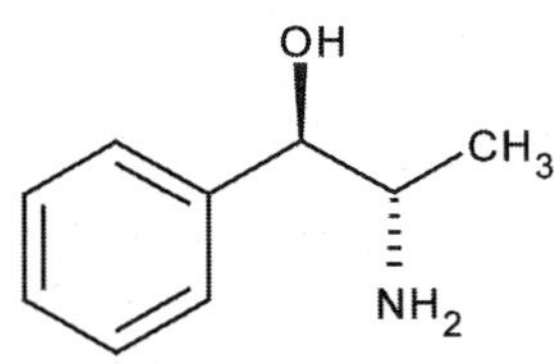

Norephedrine

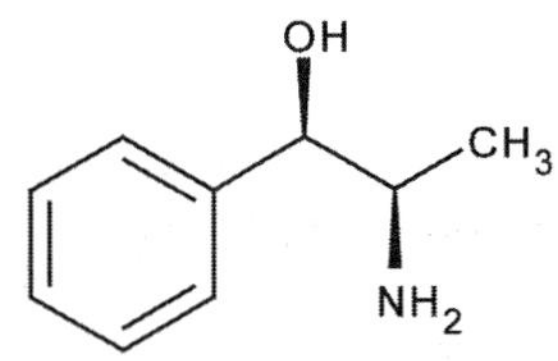

Norpseudoephedrine

Methods of Analysis

Analysis of the ephedrine alkaloids in ephedra presents a number of challenges. All six ephedrine alkaloids are structurally similar. They are hydrophilic amine compounds that have poor retention on a traditional reversed-phase HPLC system. Their basic nature often leads to excessively broad peaks and peak tailing on chromatographic systems. Lastly, they have poor UV absorption above about 210 nm. Usually, sample cleanup using solid-phase extraction is required to reduce interferences. Nevertheless, several methods have been published for the analysis of ephedrine alkaloids in dietary supplements. HPLC–UV, HPLC–MS, GC, and cation-exchange (CE) methods have all been used for the analysis of ephedra products. AOAC International recently adopted a HPLC–UV method for the analysis of ephedrine alkaloids in dietary supplements.

Method 1: The AOAC International–approved HPLC–UV method[1] for the analysis of ephedrine alkaloids in botanicals and dietary supplements uses strong cation-exchange (SCX) solid-phase extraction (SPE) as a clean-up step and short-wavelength UV detection. This method is able to separate all six ephedrine alkaloid diastereomers and to quantify ephedrine and pseudoephedrine, but it cannot separate the individual enantiomers. This method underwent a collaborative study involving 10 international laboratories. A disadvantage to this method is that caffeine has a very late eluting peak; therefore, samples that contain caffeine require a column flush with high organic concentration after every fourth injection.

Sample preparation: Prepare samples in a diluent consisting of 97% 10 mM KH_2PO_4 and 3% methanol. Treat all samples to a SPE step using a SCX column to remove interferences. Then load 5 mL of the sample solution onto a conditioned SPE cartridge and wash with 1 mL of 50 mM H_3PO_4, then with 2 mL of methanol. Elute the ephedrine alkaloids from the SPE column into a 10-mL volumetric flask with a solution of 5% NH_4OH in methanol, and dilute to volume with 500 mM H_3PO_4. An internal standard is not used.

Chromatography

Column: Phenomenex Synergi Polar RP, 150 × 4.6 mm.

Mobile phase: 3% Methanol–97% KH_2PO_4 buffer (100 mM).

Flow rate: 1.5 mL/minute

Injection volume: 20 μL

Detection wavelength: 210 nm

Run time: 20 minutes

Validation data:

Linearity: 3 to 200 mcg/mL, $r^2 > 0.9979$, recovery = 98.0% to 101%.

Accuracy: 84.6% to 98.2% recovery (two spike levels of negative control).

Repeatability: 0.98% to 2.6% RSD for ephedrine, 2.0% to 4.1% RSD for pseudoephedrine, 0.85% to 3.0% RSD for ephedrine + pseudoephedrine.

Reproducibility: 2.1% to 6.6% RSD for ephedrine, 9.0% to 11.2% RSD for pseudoephedrine, 2.0% to 7.5% RSD for ephedrine + pseudoephedrine.

Selectivity: Niacinamide was demonstrated to be a potential interferent with norpseudoephedrine.

Robustness: Not specified

LOD/LOQ: LOD = ~0.5 mcg/g of each alkaloid.

Method 2: Hurlbut et al.[2] developed a HPLC–UV method that also used SPE with a SCX cartridge for sample cleanup. This method has a detection wavelength of 255 nm, which improves selectivity but greatly reduces the sensitivity of the method. Detection limits are estimated to be approximately 0.5 mg/g.

Sample preparation: Extract about 0.5 g of sample in 25 mL of aqueous diluent. Filter the solution, and treat 1 mL of the filtrate to SPE on a CE column. Elute the ephedrine alkaloids with 4 mL of buffer containing 16.4 g of sodium acetate in 970 mL of water with 8 mL of acetic acid, 3 mL of triethylamine, and 20 mL of acetonitrile (pH 4.8). Dilute this solution to 10 mL with water.

Chromatography

Column: YMC Phenyl, 5 µm, 250 × 3.0 mm.

Mobile phase: 16.4 g of sodium acetate in 1.94 L of water with 16 mL of acetic acid, 6.0 mL of triethylamine, and 40 mL of acetonitrile.

Flow rate: 0.8 mL/minute

Injection volume: 20 µL

Detection wavelength: 255 nm

Validation data:

Linearity: 4 to 300 mcg/mL for each ephedrine alkaloid with correlation coefficients greater than 0.9999.

Accuracy: 71.5% to 102%, depending on the ephedrine alkaloid.

Precision: 1.5% to 15% RSD (ephedrine + pseudoephedrine).

Selectivity: Three herbal matrix "blanks" showed no interferences with ephedrine alkaloids.

Ruggedness: A second laboratory analyzed the same samples with good agreement with the first laboratory.

Robustness: Changes in column temperatures, flow rates, acetonitrile concentration, HPLC column lots, and SPE column lots did not significantly affect results.

LOD/LOQ: LOD = 0.5 mg of ephedrine alkaloid per g.

Method 3: Krol[3] developed a method that was considered by AOAC International for adoption. The Krol method can be considered complementary to Method 1. Krol uses a basic mobile phase (pH 9.45) requiring a column that can withstand basic conditions. The advantage to this approach is that it allows for a higher organic concentration in the mobile phase, resulting in less carryover. Caffeine elutes before the ephedrine alkaloids in this system, so a column wash is not needed for samples that contain caffeine. The disadvantage of this method is that the mobile phase is near the pK_a of the ephedrine alkaloids: small changes in pH can lead to large changes in retention time. Solid-phase extraction using a mixed-mode SPE cartridge in CE mode is performed on the samples, and 1-methyl-3-phenylpropylamine (MPPA) is used as an internal standard.

Sample preparation: Add about 1 g of sample to a 100-mL volumetric flask. Then add 20 mL of water, 50 mL of methanol, and 1 mL of internal standard solution (1000 mcg/mL MPPA) and sonicate the sample for 1 hour. Cool, and then dilute the sample to volume with methanol. Acidify 2 mL of this sample solution with 5 mL of 1% formic acid and apply to a Waters Oasis MCX cartridge (3 mL). Wash the column, in sequence, with 1 mL of 0.1 N

HCl, 1 mL of methanol, 1 mL of water, and 1 mL of 25% methanol–75% NH_4OH (5%). Elute the ephedrine alkaloids with 1.5 mL of 95% methanol–5% NH_4OH into a 5-mL volumetric flask and dilute to volume with 10 mM NH_4CO_3.

Chromatography

Column: Waters XTerra Phenyl, 3.5 µm, 150 × 2.1 mm.

Mobile phase: 10% Acetonitrile–90% 10 mM NH_4HCO_3, pH 9.45.

Flow rate: 0.23 mL/minute

Injection volume: 5 µL

Detection wavelength: 210 nm

Validation data:

Linearity: 2.5 to 250 mcg/mL for ephedrine, 2.0 to 200 mcg/mL for pseudoephedrine, 0.5 to 50 mcg/mL for the minor ephedrine alkaloids. Correlation coefficients 0.9983 to 0.9996, depending on the ephedrine alkaloid.

Accuracy: 86.9% to 121.4% average recovery, depending on the ephedrine alkaloid; from spiked matrix (Red Rose black tea).

Precision: 1.9% to 6.6% RSD for ephedrine, 4.4% to 9.8% RSD for pseudoephedrine.

Selectivity: Black tea "blank" matrix showed no interferences. In addition, selectivity was shown using UV diode-array and MS analysis.

Ruggedness: Not determined

Robustness: Not specified

LOD/LOQ: LOD $\leqq$ 10 mcg/g, LOQ $\leqq$ 50 mcg/g

Method 4: Gurley et al.[4] used ion-pair HPLC with UV detection to quantify ephedrine alkaloids in nine different products. Ion-pairing increases the retention of the ephedrine alkaloids on reversed-phase columns, increasing selectivity from other polar, nonalkaloid analytes. No SPE was performed, but an internal standard (dextroamphetamine sulfate) was incorporated. Disadvantages of the method are a long sample preparation procedure and the use of the dextroamphetamine internal standard, a DEA Schedule II controlled substance.

Sample preparation: Transfer the contents of a single tablet (crushed) or a hardshell capsule or a whole softgel to a round-bottom flask. Add 30 mL of mobile phase and reflux the contents at 80°C for 30 minutes. Centrifuge the mixture for 10 minutes at 36 × g. Decant the supernate into a 50-mL volumetric flask, and wash the residue in the centrifuge tubes with two additional 10-mL volumes of mobile phase. Add the washings to the volumetric flask, and dilute to volume with mobile phase. Transfer 500 μL of this solution to a 1.5-mL microcentrifuge tube and spike with 25 μL of internal standard solution.

Chromatography

Column: Alltech Altima C18, 5 μm, 250 × 4.6 mm.

Mobile phase: Acetonitrile–tetrahydrofuran–water (38:5:57) with 5 mM sodium lauryl sulfate.

Flow rate: 0.7 mL/minute

Injection volume: 25 μL

Detection wavelength: 208 nm

Validation data:

Linearity: 6.25 to 400 mcg/mL, correlation coefficients 0.9990 to 0.9992.

Accuracy: 92% to 99.8% recovery.

Precision: 1.6% to 6.5% intraday, depending on the alkaloid, from spiked recovery samples; 0.27% to 2.8% interday, depending on the alkaloid, from spiked recovery samples.

Selectivity: Not specified

Robustness: Not specified

LOD/LOQ: LOQ = 6.25 mcg/mL

References

1. Roman MC. Determination of ephedra alkaloids in urine and plasma by HPLC–UV: collaborative study. *J AOAC Int*. 2004 Jan–Feb;87(1):15–24.
2. Hurlbut JA, Carr JR, Singleton ER, et al. Solid-phase extraction cleanup and liquid chromatography with ultraviolet detection of ephedrine alkaloids in herbal products. *J AOAC Int*. 1998;81(6):1121–7.
3. Krol Sr J. The analysis of ephedra alkaloids at alkaline pH in botanicals and dietary supplements using LC/UV/MS. Presented at AOAC International annual meeting; September 2002; Anaheim, CA.
4. Gurley BJ, Wang P, Gardner SF. Ephedrine-type alkaloid content of nutritional supplements containing *Ephedra sinica* (Ma-huang) as determined by high-performance liquid chromatography. *J Pharm Sci*. 1998;87:1547–53.

EPIMEDIUM

Description

Botanical names: *Epimedium bravicornum* Maxim.; *Epimedium sagittatum* (Sieb.et Zucc.); *Epimedium koreanum* Nakai; *Epimedium pubescens* Maxim.; *Epimedium wushanense* T.S. Ying. These five species are listed in the Chinese Pharmacopeia as Epimedium.

Common names: Herba Epimedii, horny goat weed, Ying-Yang-Huo

Parts of plant used: Dried aerial parts

Uses: Treatment of osteoporosis and sexual dysfunctions such as impotence and seminal emission.

Mode of Action

Few clinical trials support the claims for epimedium. Any type of activity that epimedium might have was attributed to the icariin-type flavonoids. The total flavonoids extract of epimedium was found in vivo to prevent and to treat bone loss in the castrate osteoporosis rat model and to increase mineral content and to promote bone formation in mice.[1,2] Icariin, one of the major flavonoids in *Epimedium* species, was found to increase the weight of the immature mouse epididymis and seminal vesicles.[3]

Chemical Markers

Icariin-type flavonoids are believed to be main chemical components of *Epimedium*, and the major icariins are icariin, epimedin A, epimedin B, and epimedin C. Other flavonoids purified from *Epimedium* include quercetin, kaempferol-3,7-O-α-L-dirhamnoside, anhydroicaritin, ginkgetin, isoginkgetin, bilobetin, hyperoside, and 5-hydroxy-6,7-dimethyl-2,4-methylenedioxyflavone. Other compounds identified in *Epimedium* include lignans (acuminatin; icarisides E4, E5, E6, and E7; icariols A1 and A2), sterol (β-sitosterol, daucosterol, β-sitosterol glucoside), phenylethanoids (icariside, salidroside), phenylpropanoids (icariside H1), and ionone derivatives (icariside B8, icariside B9).[4–15] As icariins are the bioactive components in *Epimedium*, they are used as marker compounds for quality control; usually, four flavonoids are analyzed: icariin and epimedins A, B, and C.

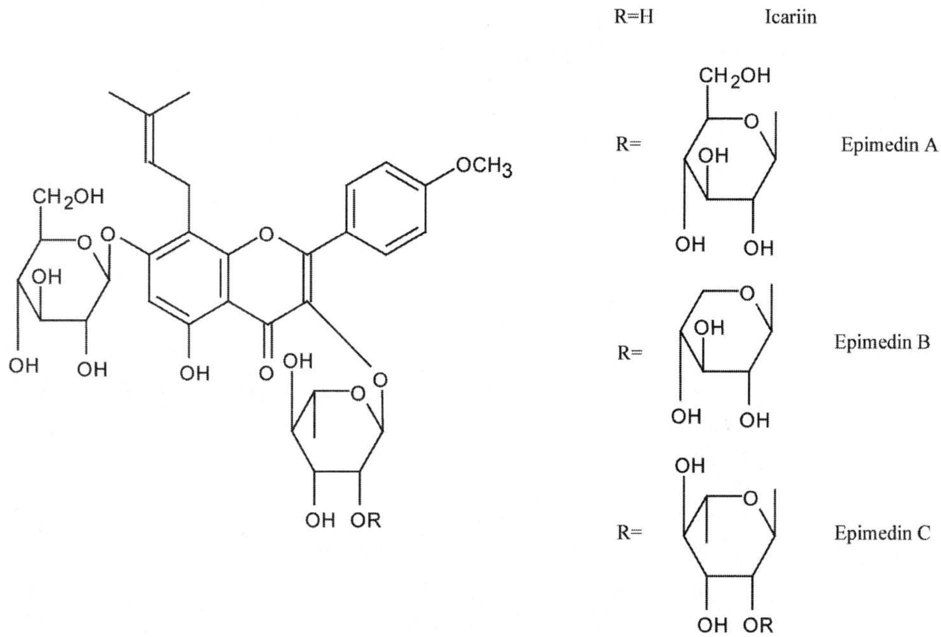

Major flavonoids in *Epimedium*.

Methods of Analysis

Icariins as flavonoids are easy to detect by UV spectrophotometry. The only challenge for the analysis of icariins is that the structures of epimedins A, B, and C are similar and it is difficult to get baseline separation.

Extraction is key for accurate analysis of icariins. Various extraction solvents have been tried including methanol, water–acetonitrile (73:27), methanol–water (50:50), ethanol–water (70:30), ethanol–water (50:50), and water combined with various extraction techniques (e.g., water bath or ultrasonication). One method uses 50% methanol as the extraction solvent, and the sample is sonicated for 30 minutes (300 mg of herbal powders in 50 mL of extraction solvent).

Method 1: The HPLC method of Ito et al.[16] was used to determine four major icariins in *Epimedium* systematically.

Sample preparation: Place about 0.5 g of dried herb powder into 25 mL of water–acetonitrile (73:27) and reflux in a water bath at 85°C for 30 minutes. Dilute the resulting extract to 50 mL with the same solvent.

Chromatography

Column: TSK gel ODS-120 Å, 5 μm, 150 × 4 mm.

Mobile phase: Water–acetonitrile (73:27) isocratic.

Flow rate: 1.0 mL/minute

Injection volume: 10 μL

Detection wavelength: 270 nm

Column temperature: 50°C

Validation data:

Linearity: 2.5 to 215.0, 5.0 to 50.0, 5.0 to 50.0, and 12.5 to 125.2 mcg for epimedins C, B, and A, and icariin, respectively, with a correlation coefficient of 0.999 for all four compounds.

Accuracy: Not specified

Precision: Not specified

Selectivity: Peak identification was determined against standards.

Ruggedness: Not specified

Robustness: Not specified

LOD/LOQ: LOD for epimedins C, B, and A and icariin were 2.5, 3, 5, and 1.3 ng/mL, respectively, at a signal-to-noise ratio of 3:1 for the peak heights.

Method 2: The method of Ma et al.[17] was used.

Sample preparation: Extract 50 mg of epimedium powder with 10 mL of methanol by sonicating for 30 minutes and shaking for 5 minutes.

Chromatography

Column: Phenomenex LiChrosorb RP-18, 5 μm, 250 × 4.6 mm.

Mobile phase: Solvent A = water, solvent B = acetonitrile.

Gradient:

Time (minutes)	%A	%B
0	80	20
20	78	22
23	75	25
35	70	30
50	50	50
55	40	60
60	0	100

Flow rate: 1.5 mL/minute

Injection volume: 10 µL

Detection wavelength: 203 nm; this method analyzes icariins and ginsenosides from ginseng at the same time.

Column temperature: 40°C

Validation data:

Linearity: Not specified

Accuracy: In the spike recovery tests, an average of 99.3% of a 1-mg icariin standard spiked into 0.25 g of epimedium extract in 10 mL of methanol was recovered.

Precision: Not specified

Selectivity: Peak identification was determined against standards.

Ruggedness: Not specified

Robustness: Not specified

LOD/LOQ: Not specified

Method 3: The unpublished method of Mingfu Wang was used.

Sample preparation: Transfer about 300 mg of epimedium powder or 50 mg of epimedium extract to a 50-mL volumetric flask, add 35 mL of extraction solvent (50% methanol), and sonicate for 30 minutes. Cool to room temperature, and fill to volume with 50% methanol.

Chromatography

Column: Phenomenex Prodigy ODS-3 100Å, 5 µm, 250 × 4.6 mm.

Mobile phase: Solvent A = water (0.2% phosphoric acid), solvent B = acetonitrile.

Gradient:

Time (minutes)	%A	%B
0	74	26
16	74	26
24	20	80
25	74	26
35	74	26

Flow rate: 1.2 mL/minute

Injection volume: 10 µL

Detection wavelength: 270 nm

Column temperature: Ambient

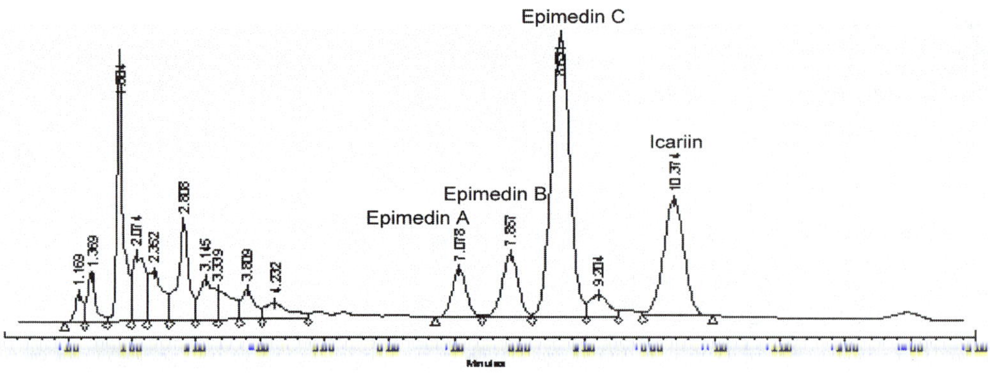

Representative HPLC chromatogram of *Epimedium koreanum* Nakai run by method 3.

References

1. Jiang Y, Mo H, Chen J. Effects of epimedium total flavonoids phytosomes on preventing and treating bone-loss of ovariectomized rats. *Zhongguo Zhong Yao Za Zhi.* 2002;27(3):221–4.
2. Yu S, Chen K, Li S, et al. *In vitro* and *in vivo* studies of the effect of a Chinese herb medicine on osteoclastic bone resorption. *Chin J Dent Res.* 1999;2(1):7–11.
3. Xiong Y, Zhou C. The effect of extracts from *Epimedium* herbs and Cuscuta seeds on male reproduction. *Zhongguo Yao Xue Za Zhi.* 1994;29(2):89–91.
4. Wu H, Lien EJ, Lien LL. Chemical and pharmacological investigations of *Epimedium* species: a survey. *Prog Drug Res.* 2003;60:1–57.
5. Han B, Shen T, Ju J, et al. Study on chemical components of *Epimedium leptorrhizum. Zhongguo Yao Xue Za Zhi.* 2002;37(5):333–5.
6. Jia X, Wu J, Mao Q. Studies on chemical constituents of *Epimedium leptorrhizum* Stearn. *Zhongguo Yao Xue Za Zhi.* 1999;34(7):442–4.
7. Sun P, Chen Y, Shimizu N, et al. Studies on the constituents of *Epimedium koreanum* Nakai. III. *Chem Pharm Bull.* 1998;46(2):355–8.
8. Yan W, Fu Y, Ma Y, et al. Studies on flavones of *Epimedium brevicorum* Maxim. *Zhongguo Zhong Yao Za Zhi.* 1998;23(12):735–6.
9. Sun P, Xu Y, Wen Y, et al. Chemical constituents of *Epimedium koreanum* Nakai. II. *Zhongguo Yaowu Huaxue Zazhi.* 1998;8(4):281–4.
10. Sun P, Xu Y, Wen Y, et al. Constituents of *Epimedium koreanum* Nakai. I. *Zhongguo Yaowu Huaxue Zazhi.* 1998;8(2):122–6.
11. Li W, Zhang R, Xiao P. Chemical constituents of Korean epimedium (*Epimedium koreanum*). *Zhong Cao Yao.* 1995;26(9):453–5.
12. Wu Q, Zhao Y, Li Z. Chemical constituents of *Epimedium sagittatum. Zhong Cao Yao.* 1995;26(9):451–2.
13. Matsushita H, Miyase T, Ueno A. Lignan and terpene glycosides from *Epimedium sagittatum. Phytochemistry.* 1991;30(6):2025–7.
14. Mizuno M, Iinuma M, Tanaka T, et al. Sutchuenoside A: a new kaempferol glycoside from the aerial parts of *Epimedium sutchuenense. J Nat Prod.* 1991;54(5):1427–9.
15. Miyase T, Ueno A, Takizawa N, et al. Ionone and lignan glycosides from *Epimedium diphyllum. Phytochemistry.* 1989;28(12):3483–5.
16. Ito Y, Hirayama F, Suto K, et al. Determination of flavonol glycosides in Epimedii Herba by high-performance liquid chromatography. *J Chromatogr A.* 1988;456(2):392–7.
17. Ma YC, Luo M, Wittenberg S, et al. Qualitative and quantitative evaluations of epimedium and ginseng combinations using HPLC. *J Chin Pharm Sci.* 2003;12(1):6–9.

FEVERFEW

Description

Botanical names: *Tanacetum parthenium* (L.) *Sch. Bip* [syn. *Chrysanthemum parthenium* (L.) Bernh.]

Common names: Bachelor's buttons, featherfew

Parts of plant used: Flowering tops, aerial parts or leaves; usually collected when the plant is flowering

Uses: Treatment of migraine headaches.

Mode of Action

A few clinical trials support the antimigraine activity of feverfew, but the mechanism is still not very clear. Extracts of feverfew were found to inhibit in vitro platelet aggregation, serotonin release, and smooth muscle cell function, which may contribute to its antimigraine activity.[1]

Chemical Markers

Sesquiterpenoid lactones (parthenolide, epoxyartemorin, artecanin, canin, santamarin) are believed to be the major chemical components in feverfew.[2,3] The occurrence of different sesquiterpene lactones was found to vary by the habitat of the plant. Flavonoids (6-hydroxykaempferol 3,6,4′-trimethyl ether, 6-hydroxykaempferol 3,6-dimethyl ether, quercetagetin 3,6-dimethyl ether, quercetagetin 3,6,4′-trimethyl ether and quercetagetin 3,6,3′-trimethyl ether, luteolin, apigenin, luteolin 7-glucuronides), melatonin, and tannins also were detected in feverfew.[4–6] The compounds identified in feverfew essential oil include camphor, chrysanthemyl acetate, camphene, and p-cymene.[7] For most varieties of feverfew, parthenolide is found to be the main sesquiterpene lactone, with the flowering tops and leaves containing the highest amounts (the stems and roots are not a good source for parthenolide). Therefore, parthenolide was selected as a chemical marker for quality control of feverfew. In Canada, it is recommended that feverfew powder must contain at least 0.2% parthenolide.

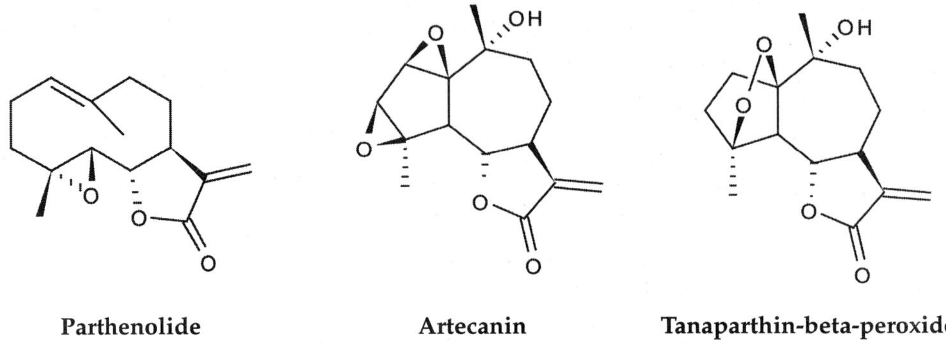

Representative sesquiterpene lactones found in feverfew.

Methods of Analysis

Most published analytical methods for the analysis of parthenolide in feverfew use reversed-phase HPLC with isocratic elution and low-wavelength detection.[1,8–10] Since parthenolide is the main chemical in feverfew, the analysis of feverfew is not very challenging and most of the published HPLC methods are good enough for parthenolide analysis. A GC method is an alternative method for parthenolide analysis.[11]

Extraction is key for accurate analysis of parthenolide in feverfew. Since parthenolide is a low polar compound, pure organic solvents such as methanol, ethanol, acetonitrile, and acetone are good extraction solvents. A small portion of water (10%, 20%, or 30%) in these solvents helps dissolve the hydrophilic components and helps the organic solvent catch parthenolide.[10] Based on the authors' experience, sonication of 250 mg of feverfew powder with 50 mL of methanol for 30 minutes is sufficient to extract parthenolide totally from feverfew.

Method 1: The method of Zhou et al. was used.[10]

Sample preparation: Various extraction solvents and extraction methods were tried; 90% acetonitrile aqueous solution was selected. The sample was prepared by bottle-stirring 1.5 g of feverfew with 100 mL of extraction solvent for 30 minutes.

Chromatography

Column: Nacalai Tesque Cosmosil C18-AR column, 5 μm, 150 × 4.6 mm, 120 Å.

Mobile phase: Acetonitrile–water (55:45) isocratic.

Flow rate: 1.5 mL/minute

Injection volume: 5 μL

Detection wavelength: 210 nm

Validation data:

Linearity: 0.16 to 850 mcg/mL with a correlation coefficient of 0.9999.

Accuracy: In the spiked recovery tests, an average of 99.3% of 7.50±0.30 mg of parthenolide standard spiked into a 0.75-g feverfew sample in 100 mL of extraction solvent was recovered with an RSD of 1.6%.

Precision: 0.88% RSD

Selectivity: Peak identification was determined against standards.

Ruggedness: Not specified

Robustness: The method was repeated on two different types of columns with comparable results.

LOD/LOQ: LOD = 0.10 ng; LOQ = 0.16 ng.

Method 2: The method of Abourashed and Khan[9] was used.

Chromatography

Column: LiChrosphere C18, 5 µm, 250 × 4.6 mm, with a SecurityGuard cartridge system (Phenomenex).

Mobile phase: Solvent A = 50 mM NaH_2PO_4 in water; solvent B = acetonitrile–methanol (90:10).

Gradient: 50%B to 85%B in 20 minutes.

Flow rate: 1.0 mL/minute

Injection volume: 20 µL

Detection wavelength: 210 nm

Validation data:

Linearity: 0 to 0.4 mg/mL with a correlation coefficient of 0.9999.

Accuracy: 103.1% recovery for parthenolide.

Precision: The RSDs with all measurements are between 0 and 3.24% (n = 3).

Selectivity: Peak identification was determined against standards.

Ruggedness: Not specified

Robustness: Not specified

LOD/LOQ: Not specified

Method 3: The unpublished method of Mingfu Wang was used.

Sample preparation: Extract a standardized extract (0.7% parthenolide) or herb powders (about 250 mg) with about 35 mL of methanol in a 50-mL volumetric flask by sonication for 30 minutes. After cooling to room temperature, fill to volume with methanol.

Chromatography

Column: Phenomenex Luna C18(2), 5 μm, 250 × 4.6 mm.

Mobile phase: Acetonitrile–water (0.2% phosphoric acid by volume) (50:50) isocratic.

Flow rate: 1.0 mL/minute

Column temperature: Ambient

Injection volume: 20 μL

Detection wavelength: 210 nm

Validation data: Not available

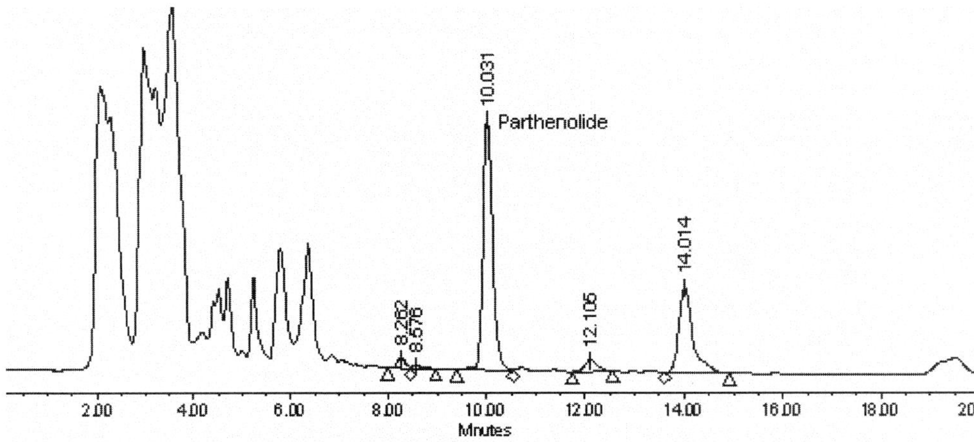

Representative HPLC chromatogram of feverfew run by method 3.

References

1. Cutlan AR, Bonilla LE, Simon JE, et al. Intra-specific variability of feverfew: correlations between parthenolide, morphological traits and seed origin. *Planta Med.* 2000;66(7): 612–7.
2. Hewlett MJ, Begley MJ, Groenewegen WA, et al. Sesquiterpene lactones from feverfew, *Tanacetum parthenium*: isolation, structural revision, activity against human blood platelet function and implications for migraine therapy. *J Chem Soc Perkin Trans I.* 1996(16):1979–86.
3. Milbrodt M, Schroeder F, Koenig WA. 3,4-β-Epoxy-8-deoxycumambrin B, a sesquiterpene lactone from *Tanacetum parthenium*. *Phytochemistry.* 1997;44(3):471–4.
4. Williams CA, Harborne JB, Geiger H, et al. The flavonoids of *Tanacetum parthenium* and *T. vulgare* and their anti-inflammatory properties. *Phytochemistry.* 1999;51(3):417–23.
5. Murch SJ, Simmons CB, Saxena PK. Melatonin in feverfew and other medicinal plants. *Lancet.* 1997;350(9091):1598–9.
6. Williams CA, Hoult JR, Harborne JB, et al. A biologically active lipophilic flavonol from *Tanacetum parthenium*. *Phytochemistry.* 1995;38(1):267–70.

7. De Pooter HL, Vermeesch J, Schamp NM. The essential oils of *Tanacetum vulgare* L. and *Tanacetum parthenium* (L.) Schultz-Bip. *J Essential Oil Res*. 1989;1(1):9–13.
8. Nelson MH, Cobb E, Shelton J. Variations in parthenolide content and daily dose of feverfew products. *Am J Health Syst Pharm*. 2002;59(16):1527–31.
9. Abourashed EA, Khan IA. Determination of parthenolide in selected feverfew products by liquid chromatography. *J AOAC Int*. 2000;83(4):789–92.
10. Zhou JZ, Kou X, Stevenson D. Rapid extraction and high-performance liquid chromatographic determination of parthenolide in feverfew (*Tanacetum parthenium*). *J Agric Food Chem*. 1999;47(3):1018–22.
11. Abourashed EA, Khan IA. GC determination of parthenolide in feverfew products. *Pharmazie*. 2001;56(12):971–2.

GINGER

Description

Botanical name: *Zingiber officinale* Roscoe

Common names: Jiang, Sunthi

Parts of plant used: Roots

Uses: Treatment of motion sickness, nausea, and osteoarthritis

Mode of Action

Ginger is one of the most important and popular spices and is used in traditional Chinese, Indian, Indonesian, and Japanese medicine. Several clinical trials have involved ginger; most showed positive effects against motion sickness, nausea, and osteoarthritis. Ginger was found to act directly at the gastric level for an antinausea effect, to reduce stimuli in the gastrointestinal tract, and to block the feedback loop between the brain stem and track.[1,2] In mechanism studies, ginger was found to inhibit prostaglandin and leukotriene synthesis and to inhibit cyclo-oxygenase and lipo-oxygenase pathways to produce anti-inflammatory effects.[3–5] Gingerols in ginger are well-known antioxidants and anti-inflammatory agents.[6,7]

Chemical Markers

Ginger rhizomes contain from 4% to 10% oleoresin. The pungent components of ginger are the gingerols with 6-gingerol (a decane substituted with a 4-hydroxy-3-methoxyphenyl group, a carbonyl group, and a hydroxyl at C-1, C-3, and C-5, respectively) as the major pungent compound. Other well-known gingerols include the 3, 4, 7, 8, 10, or 12-gingerol with a 7, 8, 11, 12, 14, or 16 carbon chain length, respectively; demethoxygingerols; 4-methylated gingerols; shogaols (6, 8, or 10-shogaol); 3,5-dihydroxy and diacetoxy derivatives of gingerols; and gingerdiones.

Two other types of unique phenolic compounds found in ginger are diarylheptanoids and cyclic diarylheptanoids. Ginger diarylheptanoids are heptanes substituted with phenyl groups at the C-1 and C-7 positions, with a similar substitution pattern as the gingerols. Cyclic diarylheptanoids in ginger usually form an additional six-member ring.[6,8,9] The compounds in ginger exist not only in free form but also as glycosides.[10,11] Recently, anthocynins were also found in many kinds of Japanese ginger, with peonidin-3-rutinoside and cyanidin-3-glucoside as the major ones.[12] The volatile ginger oil was characterized by the presence of geranial, neral, 1,8-cineole, zingiberene, β-sesquiphellandrene, ar-curcumene, and β-bisabolene by GC and GC–MS.[13,14]

The volatile oil content and the total amount of gingerols are used as quality control standards for ginger powder, oil, and extracts in the U.S. market.

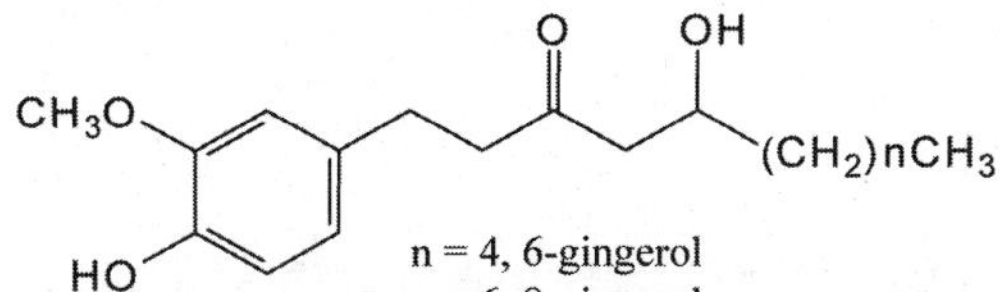

n = 4, 6-gingerol
n = 6, 8-gingerol
n = 8, 10-gingerol

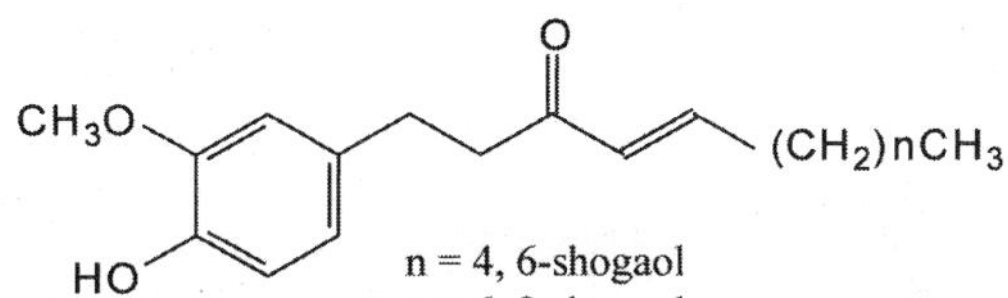

n = 4, 6-shogaol
n = 6, 8-shogaol
n = 8, 10-shogaol

Methods of Analysis

Various methods (GC–MS, HPLC, LC–MS, TLC) have been used to analyze the chemical components of ginger because ginger is such an important spice and traditional medicine. As gingerols are thermally unstable and may form many artifacts at high temperature during GC and GC–MS analysis, HPLC is the most favorable method for accurate analysis of gingerols in ginger.

Extraction is key for accurate analysis of total gingerols. As fat-soluble compounds, gingerols are easy to extract by pure methanol, acetone, and other organic solvents.

Method 1: The method found at www.nsfina.org was used.

Sample preparation: For root material, sonicate 0.4 to 0.5 g of ground material with 20 mL of methanol for 12 hours. Cool to room temperature, and bring to 25 mL with methanol.

For extracts, extract about 0.4 to 0.5 g with 20 mL of methanol for 30 minutes. Cool to room temperature, and dilute to volume with methanol.

Chromatography

Column: YMC-Pack Pro C18, 5 μm, 250 × 4.6 mm, 120 Å, or equivalent.

Mobile phase: Solvent A = water, solvent B = acetonitrile.

Gradient:

Time (minutes)	%A	%B
0	55	45
8	50	50
15	45	55
40	10	90
45	55	45
55	55	45

Flow rate: 1.0 mL/minute
Injection volume: 20 μL
Detection wavelength: 282 nm
Column temperature: 30°C

Validation data: Not available, but this method is known to be a fully validated method.

Method 2: The method of He et al.[15] was used.

Sample preparation: Grind 1 g of fresh ginger, and extract by refluxing with 20 mL of methanol for 1 hour.

For ginger oleoresin, dissolve 50 mg in 10 mL of methanol.

Chromatography
Column: Water Symmetry C18, 5 μm, 150 × 2.1 mm.
Mobile phase: Solvent A = water, solvent B = acetonitrile.
Gradient:

Time (minutes)	%A	%B
0	55	45
8	50	50
17	35	65
32	0	100
38	0	100
40	55	45

Flow rate: 0.2 mL/minute
Injection volume: 8 μL
Detection wavelength: 282 nm
Column temperature: 48°C

Validation data: Not available

Method 3: The method of Balladin et al.[16] was used.

Chromatography
Column: Ultrasphere ODS C18, 150 × 4.6 mm with a guard column (2.5 × 4.6 mm).
Mobile phase: Solvent A = water, solvent B = methanol.
Gradient: Isocratic 70%B.
Flow rate: 1.2 mL/minute

Injection volume: 20 μL
Detection wavelength: 282 nm

Validation data: Not available

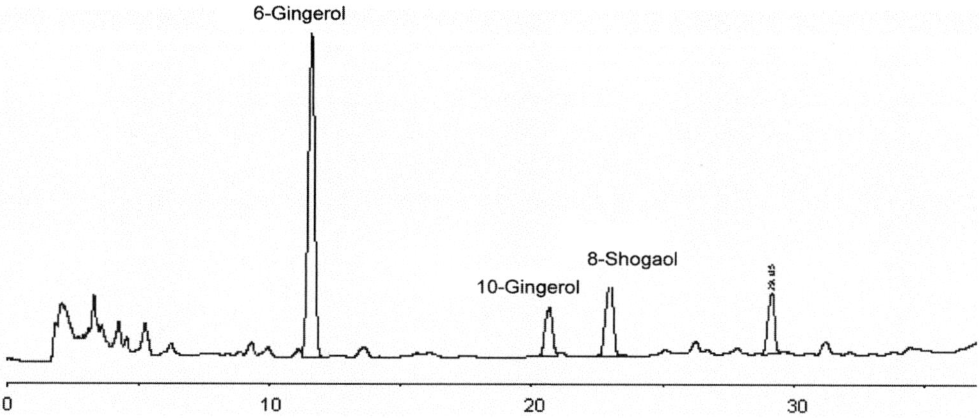

Representative HPLC chromatogram of ginger extract run by method 1 using a different HPLC column [Phenomenex Luna C18(2), 5 μm, 250 × 4.6 mm].

References

1. Holtmann S, Clarke AH, Scherer H, et al. The anti-motion sickness mechanism of ginger. A comparative study with placebo and dimenhydrinate. *Acta Otolaryngol*. 1989;108(3–4): 168–74.
2. Mowrey DB, Clayson DE. Motion sickness, ginger, and psychophysics. *Lancet*. 1982; 1(8273):655–7.
3. Thomson M, Al-Qattan KK, Al-Sawan SM, et al. The use of ginger (*Zingiber officinale* Rosc.) as a potential anti-inflammatory and antithrombotic agent. *Prostaglandins Leukot Essent Fatty Acids*. 2002;67(6):475–8.
4. Noh MS, Ha JY, Lee CH, et al. Inhibitory activities of natural products on lipopolysaccharide-induced prostaglandin production in mouse macrophages. *Yakhak Hoechi*. 1998;42(6):558–66.
5. Venkateshwarlu V. Cyclo-oxygenase inhibitors from spices. *Indian Drugs*. 1997; 34(8):427–32.
6. Nakatani N, Kikuzaki H. *Antioxidants in ginger family*. ACS symposium series 803: quality management of nutraceuticals. American Chemical Society, Washington, DC: 2002; 230–40.
7. Tjendraputra EF, Tran VH, Liu-Brennan D, et al. Effect of ginger constituents and synthetic analogues on cyclo-oxygenase-2 enzyme in intact cells. *Bioorg Chem*. 2001;29(3): 156–63.
8. He W, Li L, Li Y, et al. Antioxidative activity of a new compound from ginger. *Zhongguo Bingli Shengli Zazhi*. 2001;17(5):461–3.
9. Charles R, Garg SN, Kumar S. New gingerdione from the rhizomes of *Zingiber officinale*. *Fitoterapia*. 2000;71(6):716–8.

10. Sekiwa Y, Kubota K, Kobayashi A. Isolation of novel glucosides related to gingerdiol from ginger and their antioxidative activities. *J Agric Food Chem.* 2000;48(2):373–7.
11. Sekiwa Y, Mizuno Y, Yamamoto Y, et al. Isolation of some glucosides as aroma precursors from ginger. *Biosci Biotechnol Biochem.* 1999;63(2):384–9.
12. Iijima Y, Yoshiara M, Morimitsu Y, et al. Anthocyanin compounds in Japanese ginger (*Zingiber officinale* Roscoe) and their quantitative characteristics. *Food Sci Technol Res.* 2003;9(3):292–6.
13. Ahmad A, Naqvi AA, Aggarwal KK. Essential oil composition of different rhizomes of ginger (*Zingiber officinale* Rosc.) by GC–MS. *FAFAI J.* 2002;4(3):39–41.
14. Ekundayo O, Laakso I, Hiltunen R. Composition of ginger (*Zingiber officinale* Roscoe) volatile oils from Nigeria. *Flavour Fragrance J.* 1988;3(2):85–90.
15. He XG, Bernart MW, Lian LZ, et al. High-performance liquid chromatography–electrospray mass spectrometric analysis of pungent constituents of ginger. *J Chromatogr A.* 1998;796(2):327–34.
16. Balladin DA, Headley O, Chang-Yen I, et al. High pressure liquid chromatographic analysis of the main pungent principles of solar dried West Indian ginger (*Zingiber officinale* Roscoe). *Renewable Energy.* 1998;13(4):531–6.

GINKGO

Description

Botanical name: *Ginkgo biloba* L.

Common names: Maidenhair tree, Yin-Xing-Ye

Parts of plant used: Leaves

Uses: Treatment of poor memory, memory loss, Alzheimer's disease, peripheral vascular disease.

Mode of Action

More than 100 clinical trials have investigated the bioactivities of standardized ginkgo leaf extracts. Most of them showed effectiveness for memory loss, Alzheimer's disease, and peripheral vascular disease. The compounds responsible for the activities of ginkgo are terpene lactones and flavonol glycosides. The terpene lactones were found to inhibit platelet-activating factors, and the ginkgo flavonoids were found to act as free radical scavengers, inhibiting nitric oxide formation.

Chemical Markers

Various compounds have been identified from ginkgo leaves including terpenes, flavonoids, long-chain hydrocarbon derivatives (long-chain hydrocarbons, alcohols, aldehydes, ketones, acids), alicyclic acids and cyclic compounds (shikimic acid, quinic acid, ascorbic acid, ginkgolic acids), carbohydrates, sterols, and carotenoids. Terpene lactones and flavonoids are the major compounds in ginkgo. The terpene lactones from ginkgo have one of two characteristic skeletons: they have a diterpene structure as in ginkgolide A, B, C, J, and M, or they have a sesquiterpene structure as in bilobalide.

Ginkgo flavonoids are represented by flavonol glycosides and biflavonoids. Ginkgo leaves contain about 20 flavonol glycosides, mainly mono-, di-, and triglycosides, and p-coumarin esters of glycosides of kaempferol, quercetin, and isorhamnetin. The biflavonoids in ginkgo are all 3′,8″- biflavones (bilobetin, ginkgetin, isoginkgetin, amentoflavone, sciadopitysin, 5′-methoxybilobetin).

Ginkgo also contains other types of flavonoids including glycosides of myricetin, 3′-methyl myricetin, apigenin, luteolin, and catechins.[1,2] Currently, the content of terpene lactones (ginkgolides, bilobalide) and flavonol glycosides (glycosides of quercetin, kaempferol, and isorhamnetin) are used as the marker compounds for quality control of ginkgo leaf extract. The ginkgolic acids also are analyzed, and generally the amount of ginkgolic acids is required to be lower than 5 ppm because they are possible toxic compounds.

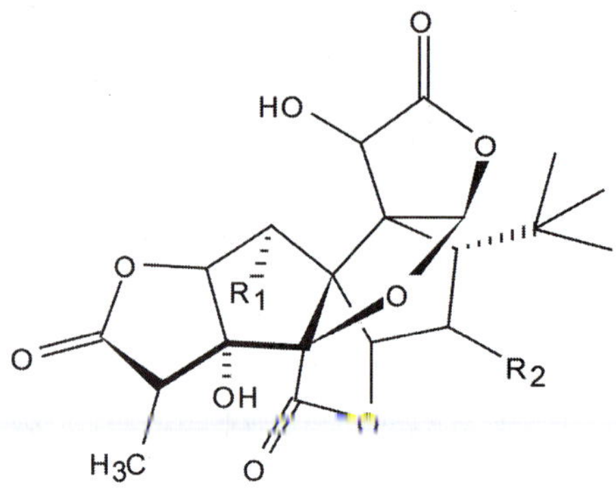

Ginkgolide A: $R_1 = H$, $R_2 = H$
Ginkgolide B: $R_1 = OH$, $R_2 = H$
Ginkgolide C: $R_1 = OH$, $R_2 = OH$
Ginkgolide J: $R_1 = H$, $R_2 = OH$

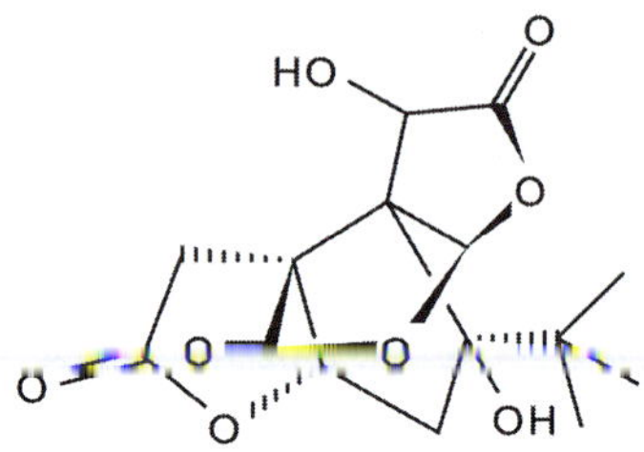

Bilobalide

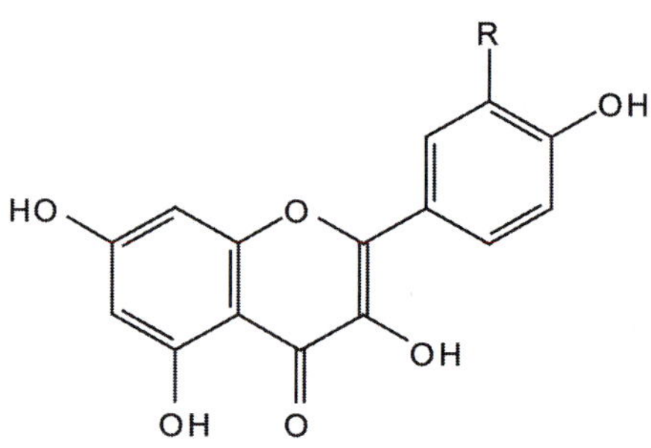

Kaempferol: R = H
Quercetin: R = OH
Isorhamnetin: R = OCH_3

Methods of Analysis

As one of the best-selling herbal medicines in the world, ginkgo has been studied extensively and reviewed by van Beek.[3] Extraction is key for accurate analysis of ginkgo compounds. Various extraction solvents have been compared for the analysis of terpene lactones; aqueous methanol, ethanol, and acetone were all found to be suitable extraction solvents. The flavonoid glycosides in ginkgo also can be extracted with aqueous alcohol.

Method 1: The method found at www.nsfina.org can be used to determine the flavonoid glycosides content in ginkgo. The glycosides are hydrolyzed with acid to produce the aglycones, kaempferol, quercetin, and isorhamnetin. The aglycones are quantified externally against pure reference standards and then converted back to glycosides using a cofactor.

Sample preparation: For plant material, accurately weigh approximately 1.0 g of ground ginkgo leaves into a 250-mL flask; add 50 mL of ethanol, 20 mL of water, and 8 mL of concentrated hydrochloric acid; and reflux at moderate heat for 2.25 hours. Decant the solution into a 100-mL volumetric flask. Add 20 mL of methanol to the hydrolysis flask, sonicate for 30 minutes at 30°C to 40°C, then transfer the solution with filtering to the 100-mL volumetric flask, and carefully wash the solids to final volume.

For extracts, weigh about 300 mg into a 250-mL flask; add 50 mL of ethanol, 20 mL of water (deionized, distilled), and 8 mL of concentrated hydrochloric acid; sonicate for 5 minutes; and reflux at moderate heat for 2.25 hours. Dilute the extraction solution to 100 mL.

Chromatography

Column: Phenomenex Prodigy ODS(3), 5 μm, 100Å, 250 × 4.6 mm.

Mobile phase: Methanol–0.5% phosphoric acid (50:50), isocratic.

Flow rate: 1.2 to 1.5 mL/minute

Injection volume: 10 μL

Column temperature: 35°C

Detection wavelength: 270 nm

Correction factors for conversion of the aglycone to the glycoside:

For quercetin, F = 756.7/302.2 = 2.504.

For kaempferol, F = 740.7/286.2 = 2.588.

For isorhamnetin, F = 770.6/316.2 = 2.437.

Method 2: The method at www.nsfina.org also can be used to analyze the terpene lactones in ginkgo.

Sample preparation: For plant materials, accurately weigh 600 to 800 mg into a 50-mL round-bottom flask fitted with a reflux condenser. Reflux with 5 mL of methanol–water (90:10) for 15 minutes. Filter the sample through a Büchner funnel and extract the leaf material with another 5 mL of methanol–water (90:10). Filter and combine the collected filtrates and washes, then dry under a stream of nitrogen. Finally, dissolve the residues in 1 mL of methanol for HPLC analysis.

For the extract, weigh approximately 400 mg into a 50-mL volumetric flask along with 40 mL of methanol–water (90:10). Sonicate at 60°C for 20 minutes or until completely dissolved. Filter the solution before HPLC analysis.

Chromatography

Column: Phenomenex Prodigy ODS(3), 5 μm, 100Å, 250 × 4.6 mm.

Mobile phase: Solvent A = water, solvent B = methanol.

Gradient:

Time (minutes)	%A	%B
0	75	25
23	52	48
25	25	75
30	25	75
35	10	90
40	75	25
50	75	25

Column temperature: 25°C
Flow rate: 1.0 mL/minute
Injection volume: 8 µL
Detector: ELSD

Method 3: The HPLC method of Ganzera et al.[4] was used for the analysis of terpene lactones (ginkgolides A, B, C, and J and bilobalide) in ginkgo.

Sample preparation: Extract about 500 mg of sample three times with 3 mL of methanol by sonication for 10 minutes. Centrifuge after each extraction and combine the supernates. Fill to 10 mL with methanol.

Chromatography

Column: Phenomenex Synergi Max RP, 80Å, 4 µm, 150 × 4.6 mm.

Mobile phase: Solvent A = 10 mM ammonium acetate buffer adjusted to pH 5 with glacial acetic acid, solvent B = methanol–isobutanol (9:1).

Gradient: in 10 minutes from 10%B to 20%B, then to 25%B in 15 minutes.

Flow rate: 1.0 mL/minute

Injection volume: 20 µL

Column temperature: 25°C

Detection wavelength: 205 nm and ELSD detector

Validation data:

Linearity: 31.2 to 500 mcg/mL with a correlation coefficient of 0.9988 for all five compounds.

Accuracy: 98.26% and 100.10% recovery for bilobalide and ginkgolide J, respectively.

Precision: 3.07% RSD (three determinations)

Selectivity: Peak identification was determined against standards.

Ruggedness: Not specified

Robustness: Not specified

LOD/LOQ: Between 10 and 20.3 mcg/mL for five standards.

Method 4: Another analytical method is that of Li and Fitzloff.[5]

Sample preparation: Extract five units (capsules, tablets, or caplets) with 25 mL of 80% methanol through sonication for 60 minutes, then extract two more times with 25 mL of 80% methanol and sonicate 30 minutes each time. Combine the extraction solutions and evaporate under reduced pressure. Dissolve the residue in 50 mL of 80% methanol.

For total flavonoid analysis, reflux 5 mL of the sample preparation solution with 25 mL of hydrochloric acid (4 N)–methanol (1:4 vol/vol) for 30 minutes. Cool, then make up to 50 mL with methanol.

For terpene lactone analysis, evaporate 10 mL of the sample preparation solution to dryness, suspend the residue in 20 mL of hot water, and extract with acetyl acetate (3 × 20 mL). Evaporate the acetyl acetate to dryness and dissolve the residue in 10 mL of methanol.

Chromatography

Column: Supelco Discovery RP-18, 5 µm, 250 × 4.6 mm, with a Waters Delta-Pak RP-18 guard column.

Mobile phase: Solvent A = water (5% methanol and 0.05% trifluoroacetic acid), solvent B = methanol (0.05% trifluoroacetic acid). For flavonoid analysis, mobile phase is 50%B isocratic for 20 minutes.

Column temperature: 20°C

Detection wavelength: 365 nm

Injection volume: 10 µL

Flow rate: Not specified

For terpene lactone analysis, mobile phase is 25%B to 50%B in 20 minutes.

Injection volume: 10 µL

Flow rate: Not specified

Detector: ELSD

Validation data:

Linearity: For quercetin, kaempferol, and isorhamnetin, 4 to 2000 mcg/mL with correlation coefficient over 0.9953; for ginkgolide A, B, and C and bilobalide, 40 to 2000 mcg/mL with a correlation coefficient over 0.9975; and for ginkgolide J, 70 to 3500 mcg/mL with a correlation coefficient over 0.9992.

Accuracy: For quercetin, kaempferol, and isorhamnetin, over 97.55% recovery; and for bilobalide, ginkgolide A, B, C, and J, between 93.24% and 97.91%.

Precision: Less than 3.77% for all eight standards.

Selectivity: Peak identification was determined against standards.

Ruggedness: Not specified

Robustness: Not specified

LOD/LOQ: LOD for quercetin, kaempferol, isorhamnetin, ginkgolide A, B, C, and J, and bilobalide = 2, 2, 2, 20, 20, 20, 35, and 20 ng, respectively. LOQ for quercetin, kaempferol, isorhamnetin, ginkgolide A, B, C, J, and bilobalide = 4, 4, 4, 40, 40, 40, 70, and 40 ng, respectively.

Method 5: The method of Fuzzati et al.[6] can be used to analyze ginkgolic acids in ginkgo extract.

Sample preparation: Dissolve 500 mg of ginkgo solution in 10 mL of methanol.

Chromatography

Column: Agilent Zorbax Eclipse XDB-C8, 5 μm, 250 × 4.6 mm.

Mobile phase: Solvent A = water (0.01% trifluoroacetic acid), solvent B = acetonitrile.

Gradient:

Time (minutes)	%A	%B
0	25	75
30	10	90
35	10	90

Flow rate: 1 mL/minute

Detection wavelength: 210 nm

Column temperature: 35°C

Injection volume: 50 μL

Validation data:

Linearity: For ginkgolic acid C13, 0.05 to 2 mcg/mL; for ginkgolic acid C15, 0.15 to 8 mcg/mL; and for ginkgolic acid C17, 0.06 to 3 mcg/mL. The correlation coefficient was over 0.999 for all.

Accuracy: All recovery values were between 82.5% and 121.2%.

Precision: RSDs were between 0.1% and 9.0%.

Selectivity: Peak identification was determined against standards.

Ruggedness: Not specified

Robustness: Not specified

LOD/LOQ: LOD = About 0.025 mcg/mL for all three compounds; LOQ = about 0.083 mcg/mL for all three compounds.

References

1. Sticher O. Ginkgo preparation: biochemical, pharmaceutical and medical perspectives. In: Kanba S, Richelson E, eds. *Herbal medicines for neuropsychiatric diseases, current developments and research*. Seiwa Shoten Publishers and Brunner/Mazel; 1999:83–115.
2. Bruneton J. *Pharmacognosy, Phytochemistry, Medicinal plants*. Paris: Lavoisier Publishing; 1995:282–3.
3. Van Beek TA. Chemical analysis of *Ginkgo biloba* leaves and extracts. *J Chromatogr A*. 2002;967(1):21–55.
4. Ganzera M, Zhao J, Khan IA. Analysis of terpene lactones in *Ginkgo biloba* by high-performance liquid chromatography and evaporative light-scattering detection. *Chem Pharm Bull*. 2001;49(9):1170–3.
5. Li W, Fitzloff JF. HPLC determination of flavonoids and terpene lactones in commercial *Ginkgo biloba* products. *J Liq Chromatogr Relat Technol*. 2002;25(16):2501–14.
6. Fuzzati N, Pace R, Villa F. A simple HPLC–UV method for the assay of ginkgolic acids in *Ginkgo biloba* extracts. *Fitoterapia*. 2003;74(3):247–56.

GINSENG

Description

Botanical names: *Panax ginseng; Panax quinquefolium*

Common names: American ginseng (*Panax quinquefolium*), Asian ginseng, Chinese ginseng (*Panax ginseng*), Korean ginseng

NOTE: *Eleutherococcus senticosus* (Eleuthero) is often referred to as "Siberian ginseng"; however, it is not related to Asian or American ginseng, and the following analytical methods do not apply to Eleuthero.

Parts of plant used: Roots

NOTE: Some ground ginseng powders or extracts may be adulterated with ginseng leaves. This type of adulteration usually can be detected by visual inspection: the material will have a green tint, as opposed to the typical reddish brown tint obtained from the roots.

Uses: Both Asian and American ginsengs traditionally have been used as tonics to reduce effects of stress, to counteract fatigue, and to increase stamina.

Mode of Action

There is very little clinical evidence that Asian and American ginsengs possess the pharmacological properties ascribed to them. Any activity that ginseng may have is generally attributed to a group of triterpenoid saponin glycosides commonly called ginsenosides. There are two main groups of ginsenosides, which are referred to as panaxadiols or panaxatriols, depending upon the number of hydroxyl groups attached to the saponin backbone. The ginsenosides are structurally related to sterols such as cholestanol. There is no known mode of action for the ginsenosides.

Chemical Markers

Both Asian and American ginsengs are assayed for their ginsenoside content. More than 20 ginsenosides have been identified, but typically only seven are assayed: ginsenosides Rb1, Rb2, Rc, Rd, Re, Rf, and Rg1. The remaining ginsenosides are present in very low concentrations. While both Asian and American ginsengs contain these same ginsenosides, the individual ratios are different between the two species. The structures of the marker compounds follow.

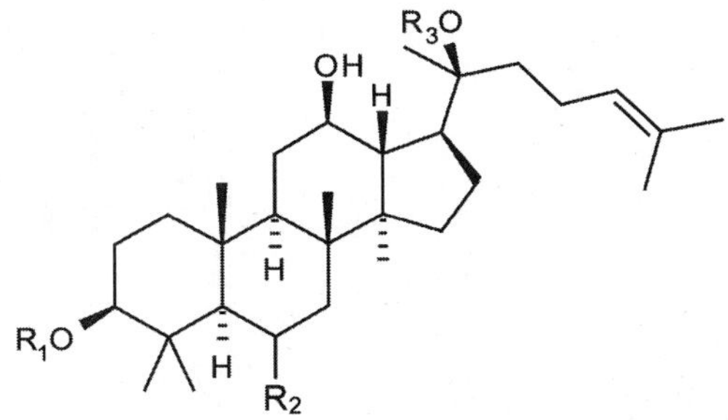

Ginsenoside	R_1	R_2	R_3
Rb1	Glc²-Glc	H	Glc⁶-Glc
Rb2	Glc²-Glc	H	Glc⁶-Ara(p)
Rc	Glc²-Glc	H	Glc⁶-Ara(f)
Rd	Glc²-Glc	H	Glc
Re	H	O-Glc²-Rha	Glc
Rf	H	O-Glc²-Glc	H
Rg1	H	O-Glc	Glc

Methods of Analysis

Most published analytical methods use reversed-phase HPLC with gradient elution and low-wavelength UV detection. Ginsenosides are very water soluble, owing to the presence of the sugar-group moieties; therefore, mobile phases are generally highly aqueous. Because ginsenosides do not possess a good chromophore, low-wavelength UV detection (203 to 205 nm) usually is used to take advantage of the absorptivity of the alkene group. Acetonitrile must be used as the organic modifier in the mobile phase to enable detection at these low wavelengths. Other more exotic detection techniques that are not dependent upon chromophores, such as evaporative light-scattering detection or MS, can be used.

Extraction of the ginsenosides from the matrix is of key importance. Ginsenosides have good solubility in aqueous extraction solvents, with decreasing solubility as the concentration of the organic modifier increases. Above about 40% organic concentration in the extraction solvent, incomplete recovery or inconsistent results occur, and multiple extractions must be performed on the sample. Acidic or basic extraction solvents also should be avoided, as hydrolysis of the glycosides can occur.

Method 1: Court et al.[1] developed a gradient reversed-phase HPLC method for the determination of not only the seven listed ginsenosides, but also ginsenosides Rg2, Ro, F11, and gypenoside XVII in ground ginseng.

Sample preparation: Extract about 300 mg of ground ginseng root with 10 mL of methanol–water (70:30) in an ultrasonication bath for 15 minutes. Remove the solvent, and repeat the extraction of the residue twice. Dry the combined extracts under vacuum, and dissolve the residue in 2 mL of water containing m-cresol internal standard.

Chromatography

Column: Waters Resolve C18, 150 × 3.9 mm, equipped with Symmetry C18 guard column.

Mobile phase: Solvent A = phosphate buffer, pH 5.81; solvent B = acetonitrile; solvent C = water.

Gradient:

Time (minutes)	%A	%B	%C
0–15	81–79	19–21	0
15–24.5	79–73.7	21–26.3	0
24.5–29	73.7–73	26.3–27	0
29–43	73–66	27–34	0
43–47	66–64	34–36	0
47–54	64–57	36–43	0
54–55	57–0	43–85	0–15
55–59	0	85	15

Flow rate: 1.15 mL/minute

Injection volume: 5 μL

Detection wavelength: 203 nm

Validation data:

Linearity: Not specified

Accuracy: Not specified

Precision: 1.1% to 8.7% RSD, depending on ginsenoside (six determinations).

Selectivity: Peak identification of Rb1, Rb2, Rc, Rd, Re, Rf, and Rg1 was determined against standards. In addition, selectivity was confirmed by comparing results with those obtained using a different chromatographic system.

Ruggedness: Not specified

Robustness: Not specified

LOD/LOQ: Not specified

Method 2: The Institute for Nutraceutical Advancement (INA) developed a reversed-phase gradient HPLC method[2] for the determination of ginsenosides in ginseng roots and extracts.

Sample preparation: Extract a standardized extract (about 90 mg) or ground root (about 800 mg) with 25 mL of ethanol–water (50:50) by sonicating and shaking at 50°C. Cool, add about 10 mL of acetonitrile, and dilute the sample to 50 mL with water.

Chromatography
Column: YMC ODS-A, 3.0 µm, 150 × 3 mm.
Mobile phase: Solvent A = water, solvent B = acetonitrile.
Gradient:

Time (minutes)	%A	%B
0–22	80–78	20–22
22–40	78–50	22–50
40–50	50–45	50–55
50–52	45–35	55–65

Flow rate: 0.6 mL/minute
Injection volume: 12 µL
Detection wavelength: 205 nm

Validation data:

Linearity: 0.5 to 60 mcg/mL for each ginsenoside; correlation coefficient 0.99978 to 1.00000, depending on ginsenoside. RSD of response factors: 3.37% to 9.61%, depending on ginsenoside.

Accuracy: Ginseng extracts and root material were spiked with a ginseng extract of known ginsenoside content at the 150% and 200% target. The percent recoveries were calculated and ranged from 98.5 to 106.3.

Precision: 1.47% RSD for extract sample (total ginsenosides; six determinations). 1.74% RSD for root sample (total ginsenosides; six determinations).

Selectivity: Peak identification of Rb1, Rb2, Rc, Rd, Re, Rf, and Rg1 was determined against standards. In addition, selectivity was shown using UV diode-array analysis.

Ruggedness: Three different laboratories analyzed six sets of samples. The percent RSD between the three laboratories for each sample was: Sample 1 = 5.6%; Sample 2 = 2.1%; Sample 3 = 4.6%; Sample 4 = 5.3%; Sample 5 = 5.0%; and Sample 6 = 0.7%.

Robustness: Not determined

LOD/LOQ: LOD = 0.348 to 1.58 mcg/mL, depending on the ginsenoside; LOQ = 1.16 to 5.27 mcg/mL, depending on the ginsenoside.

Method 3: Li and Fitzloff [3] developed an HPLC method with evaporative light-scattering detection (ELSD) to overcome the limitations of poor sensitivity associated with low-wavelength UV detection.

Sample preparation: Extract about 0.5 g of ground root with three 15-mL portions of methanol in a 50-mL volumetric flask using sonication and shaking at 25°C to 30°C for 30 minutes. Combine the methanol extracts and dry. Reconstitute the residue in methanol, and bring to volume in a 10-mL volumetric flask.

Chromatography

Column: Waters Spherisorb ODS-2, 5 μm, 250 × 4.6 mm.

Mobile phase: Solvent A = water, solvent B = acetonitrile.

Gradient:

Time (minutes)	%A	%B
0–20	80	20
20–60	80–58	20–42
60–61	58–10	42–90

Flow rate: 1.6 mL/minute

Injection volume: 10 μL

Detection: Sedex 75 ELSD; evaporation chamber temperature = 35°C; nebulizing gas pressure = 3.4 bar.

Validation data:

Linearity: 20 to 200 mcg/mL for each ginsenoside; correlation coefficient 0.9976 to 0.9998, depending on the ginsenoside.

Accuracy: No spiking studies were performed.

Precision: 4.23% to 9.89% CV, depending on ginsenosides; three determinations, control sample.

Selectivity: Peak identification of Rb1, Rb2, Rc, Rd, Re, Rf, and Rg1 was determined against standards. In addition, selectivity was shown using UV diode-array analysis.

Ruggedness: Not determined

Robustness: Not specified

LOD/LOQ: LOD = 50 ng for each ginsenoside; LOQ = not specified.

Method 4: Gomez-Serranillos et al.[4] developed a rapid, sensitive HPLC–UV method with solid-phase extraction (SPE) sample cleanup. The SPE step removes many interfering peaks, increasing the sensitivity of the method while allowing for a shorter run time.

Sample preparation: Extract ground ginseng root sample or powdered ginseng tablets with methanol–water (70:30) at room temperature for 30 minutes. Evaporate the solution, and reconstitute the residue in water. Apply a portion of the aqueous solution to a Waters Sep-Pak C18 cartridge. Wash the cartridge with water, and follow by methanol–water (30:70). Elute the ginsenosides with methanol. Evaporate the eluate, and reconstitute the residue with methanol–water (30:70).

Chromatography

Column: Hypersil ODS, 5 μm, 200 × 4.6 mm.

Mobile phase: Solvent A = water–acetonitrile (90:10), solvent B = acetonitrile.

Gradient:

Time (minutes)	%A	%B
0–20	75–50	25–50

Flow rate: 2.0 mL/minute

Injection volume: 10 μL

Detection wavelength: 205 nm

Validation data:

Linearity: Not specified

Accuracy: Not specified

Precision: Not specified

Selectivity: Peak identification of Rb1, Rb2, Rc, Rd, Re, Rf, and Rg1 was made against standards. In addition, selectivity was shown using UV diode-array analysis.

Ruggedness: Not specified

Robustness: The method was tried on three different brands of C18 columns with comparable results.

LOD/LOQ: Not specified

References

1. Court WA, Hendel JG, Elmi J. Reversed-phase high-performance liquid chromatographic determination of ginsenosides in *Panax quinquefolium*. *J Chromatogr A*. 1996;755:11–7.
2. Institute for Nutraceutical Advancement. Panax and American ginseng assay by HPLC. Available at: http://www.nsf.org/business/ina/index.asp?program=INA.
3. Li WK, Fitzloff JF. HPLC analysis of ginsenosides in the roots of Asian ginseng (*Panax ginseng*) and North American ginseng (*Panax quinquefolium*) with in-line photodiode array and evaporative light-scattering detection. *J Liq Chromatogr Relat Technol*. 2002; 25(1):29–41.
4. Gomez-Serranillos MP, Palomino OM, Carretero E, et al. A new HPLC method for the analysis of ginsenosides in *Panax ginseng*. *Fitoterapia*. 1997;68(6):533–6.

GLUCOSAMINE

Description

Chemical names: 2-Amino-2-deoxy-D-glucose; (2R,3R,4R,5S,6R)-3-amino-6-hydroxymethyl-tetrahydropyran-2,4,5-triol

Common name: Chitosamine

Molecular weight: 179.17

Chemical formula: $C_6H_{13}NO_5$

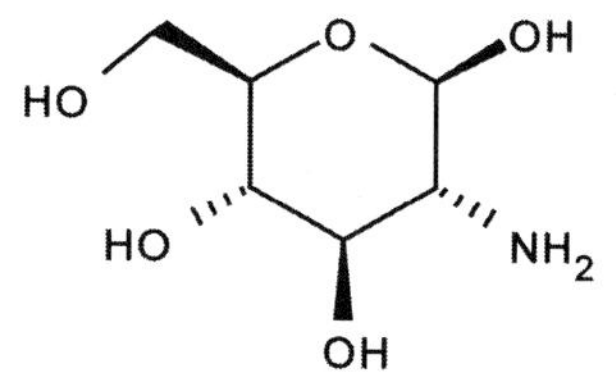

Glucosamine

Solubility: Highly water soluble; slightly soluble in cold methanol and ethanol; insoluble in ether, chloroform, benzene, and other nonpolar organic solvents.

Other physical/chemical data:

β-Form: $[\alpha]_D$ = +28° at 20°C (c = 1); melting point = 110°C (decomposition)

α-Form: $[\alpha]_D$ = +100° at 20°C (c = 1)

NOTE: Both α- and β-forms change to $[\alpha]_D$ +47.5° over time.

Uses: Glucosamine has been used to reduce the pain associated with osteoarthritis, a condition that causes progressive breakdown of the cartilage in joints. It is usually available commercially as either the hydrochloride or sulfate salt. Glucosamine is sometimes combined with chondroitin sulfate in dietary supplements.

Mode of Action

The mode of action of glucosamine is not completely understood. It seems to be related to the biosyntheses or activation of glycosaminoglycans.[1,2]

Methods of Analysis

Glucosamine is a highly polar molecule lacking a UV chromophore. As a result, methods of analysis usually involve either precolumn derivatization followed by reversed-phase HPLC or ion-exchange or ion-pair chromatography followed by either refractive index (RI) or electrochemical (EC) detection.

Although the mode of action and efficacy of glucosamine hydrochloride and glucosamine sulfate are believed to be the same, the potency is not due to the differences in molar weight between the two forms. Glucosamine free base constitutes 83.1% by weight of glucosamine hydrochloride, whereas it constitutes only 78.5% by weight of the hemisulfate form, and this amount may be even less as the hemisulfate salt often contains potassium chloride as well. Specifications and labels of glucosamine products should be examined to determine if the product is the free base or one of the salts.

Method 1: The Institute for Nutraceutical Advancement (INA) has developed a method[3] for the analysis of glucosamine in raw materials using precolumn derivatization with phenylisothiocyanate followed by reversed-phase HPLC. This method can be adapted easily to finished products containing glucosamine.

Standard and sample preparation: Weigh about 40 mg of glucosamine standard or sample (calculated as the free base), transfer to a 50-mL volumetric flask, and dissolve in 0.1 M sodium acetate solution. Pipet 5 mL of this solution into a 50-mL volumetric flask, and add 400 µL of phenylisothiocyanate and 15 mL of methanol. Fill to volume with methanol–water (60:40), and transfer 5 mL of this solution to a reaction vial, cap, and heat at 80°C for 15 minutes. Cool, and extract the solution with 5 mL of hexane to remove unreacted phenylisothiocyanate.

Chromatography

Column: Phenomenex Luna, C18, 5 µm, 150 × 4.6 mm.

Mobile phase: Acetonitrile–water–phosphoric acid (10:90:0.1).

Flow rate: 1.5 mL/minute

Injection volume: 10 µL

Detection wavelength: UV at 240 nm

Run time: 10 minutes

Validation data: Not available

Method 2: Way et al.[4] developed an ion-pair HPLC method using refractive index detection for the determination of glucosamine in dietary supplements.

Sample preparation: Weigh an amount of sample equivalent to about 100 mg of glucosamine into a 100-mL volumetric flask, and dilute to volume with mobile phase. Sonicate the samples for approximately 20 minutes to dissolve the glucosamine.

Chromatography

Column: Metachem Inertsil, ODS-3, 5 μm, 250 × 4.6 mm.

Mobile phase: 10% methanol–90% 0.005 M octanesulfonate, pH 2.1.

Flow rate: 1.0 mL/minute

Injection volume: 50 μL

Detection: Refractive index at 40°C

Validation data:

Linearity: Correlation coefficient >0.999 (52% to 210% of target).

Accuracy: Average recovery = 98.4%.

Precision: 2.13% RSD of 12 sample preparations.

Selectivity: Interferences in placebo <1% of target, verified by PDA.

Ruggedness: Average results on second day were 97.5% of first-day results.

Robustness: Not specified

LOD/LOQ: Not specified

Method 3: Another method using precolumn derivatization with phenylisothiocyanate followed by reversed-phase HPLC was developed by Liang et al.[5] The method differs from the INA method in both sample preparation and chromatography.

Standard and sample preparation: Prepare glucosamine standard solutions in water at concentrations ranging from about 6.6 to 16.6 mcg/mL. Prepare samples in water so that the glucosamine concentration is within the linearity range. To these solutions, add 250 μL of 0.3 M phosphate buffer (pH 8.0) and 250 μL of 5% phenylisothiocyanate. Incubate the solutions at room temperature for 10 minutes, and then evaporate to dryness at 50°C under nitrogen. Reconstitute the samples and standards in 200 μL of mobile phase.

Chromatography

Column: Phenomenex Bondclone C18, 10 μm, 300 × 3.9 mm.

Mobile phase: Methanol–water–acetic acid (10:89.96:0.04).

Flow rate: 1.2 mL/minute

Injection volume: 20 μL

Detection wavelength: UV at 254 nm

Run time: 10 minutes

Validation data:

Linearity: Correlation coefficient >0.99 (6.65 to 16.63 mcg/mL).

Accuracy (intraday): +0.90% to 2.54% relative error.

Accuracy (interday): 0.75% to 2.70% relative error.

Precision (intraday): 0.47% to 4.18% RSD.
Precision (interday): 0.99% to 3.18% RSD.
Selectivity: Not specified
Robustness: Determined using two different lots of the same analytical column and two different batches of mobile phase (only retention times compared).
LOD/LOQ: Not determined

References

1. Lippiello L, Woodward J, Karpman R, et al. Beneficial effect of cartilage disease-modifying agents testing in chondrocyte cultures and a rabbit instability model of osteoarthritis. *Arthritis Rheum.* 1999;42(Suppl.):S256.
2. Runkel DR, Cupp MJ. Glucosamine sulfate use in osteoarthritis. *Am J Health Syst Pharm.* 1999;56:267.
3. Institute for Nutraceutical Advancement method 121.000, panax and American ginseng assay by HPLC. http://www.nsfina.org/business/ina/index.asp?program=INA.
4. Way WK, Gibson KG, Breite AG. Determination of glucosamine in nutritional supplements by reversed-phase ion-pairing HPLC. *J Liq Chromatogr Relat Technol.* 2000;23(18): 2831–71.
5. Liang Z, Leslie J, Adebowale A, et al. Determination of the nutraceutical, glucosamine hydrochloride, in raw materials, dosage forms and plasma using pre-column derivatization with ultraviolet HPLC. *J Pharm Biomed Anal.* 1999;20:807–14.

GOLDENSEAL

Description

Botanical name: *Hydrastis canadensis* L.

Common names: Eye-balm, goldenseal, ground raspberry, wild turmeric, yellow eye, yellow paint, yellow root

Parts of plant used: Dried rhizomes and roots

Uses: Treatment of infection; inflammation; congestion of lungs, throat, and sinuses; diarrhea; colds; and flu. Immune system booster.

Mode of Action

Although goldenseal is a well-known herbal medicine in North America, it has not been evaluated in many clinical trials. There is a general belief that the major alkaloids berberine, β-hydrastine, canadine (tetrahydroberberine), and canadaline are the bioactive components in goldenseal and are responsible for its bioactivity.

Chemical Markers

The isoquinoline alkaloids are the major chemical components in goldenseal root. The total content of alkaloids in goldenseal root is about 5% and the main alkaloids are berberine, hydrastine, canadine (tetrahydroberberine), and canadaline.[1] Goldenseal also contains 8-oxotetrahydrothalifendine, canadinic acid, hydrastidine, isohydrastidine, 5-O-feruloylquinic acid butyl ester, 4-O-feruloylquinic acid butyl ester, chlorogenic acid, polyphenols, and fatty acids.[2–7] When the volatile components of goldenseal were analyzed by GC–MS, several compounds including 2,3-dihydro-3,5-dihydro-6-methyl-4H-pyran-4-none and 5-(hydroxymethyl)-2-furane carboxaldehyde were identified.[8] Usually hydrastine and berberine are used as chemical markers for quality control of goldenseal.

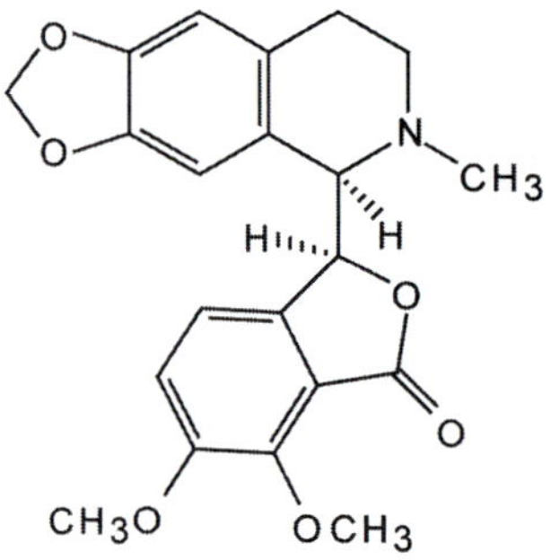

Hydrastine

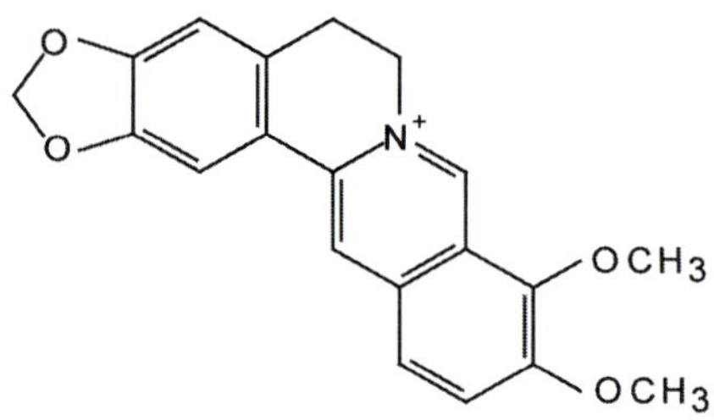

Berberine

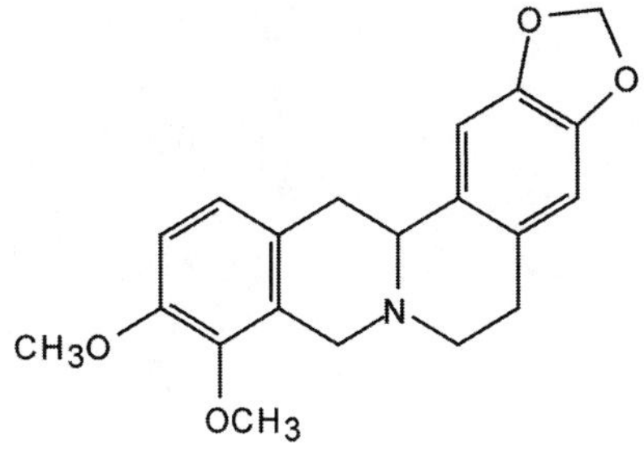

Canadine

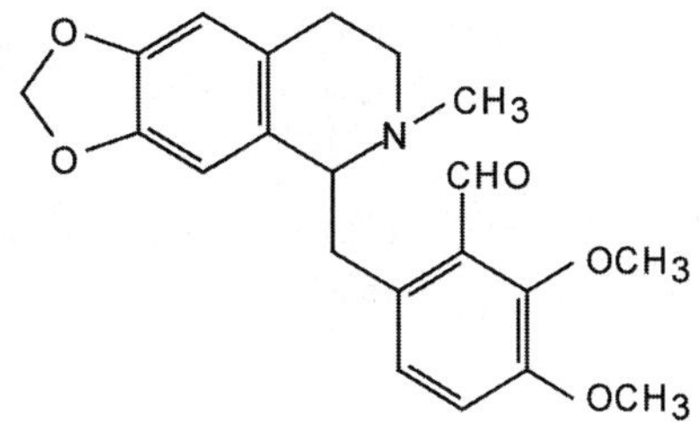

Canadaline

Methods of Analysis

HPLC is the primary method for the analysis of berberine and hydrastine in goldenseal root. Other methods include capillary electrophoresis–MS, TLC, and colorimetry.

Various extraction solvents have been used to extract alkaloids from goldenseal including methanol, 90% methanol, 70% methanol, and 50% methanol acidic solution. Based on the literature, they all extract berberine and hydrastine from goldenseal.

Method 1: The HPLC method of Abourashed and Khan[9] was used to determine the hydrastine and berberine content in powders, capsules, and tablets.

Sample preparation: Sonicate 100 mg of powder in 3 mL of methanol for 15 minutes, then centrifuge for 5 minutes at 1500 rpm. Transfer the supernate to a 10-mL volumetric flask, and repeat this procedure twice. Combine the supernates and dilute to 10 mL for HPLC analysis.

Chromatography

Column: Phenomenex Luna C18, 5 µm, 150 × 4.6 mm, and SecurityGuard cartridge system.

Mobile phase: Solvent A = 0.10 M sodium acetate–acetic acid (pH 4.0 in water), solvent B = acetonitrile–methanol (90:10).

Gradient:

Time (minutes)	%A	%B
0	80	20
20	40	60

Flow rate: 1.0 mL/minute

Injection volume: 10 µL

Detection wavelength: 290 nm

Validation data:

Linearity: 3.1 to 100 mcg/mL with a correlation coefficient of over 0.999 for berberine and hydrastine.

Accuracy: The percent recoveries were 98.38 and 98.36 for hydrastine and berberine, respectively.

Precision: 2.67% RSD for hydrastine and 0.86% RSD for berberine.

Selectivity: Peak identification was determined against standards.

Ruggedness: Not specified

Robustness: Not specified

LOD/LOQ: LOD = 1.0 mcg/mL for both compounds; LOQ = 3.13 mcg/mL for both compounds.

Method 2: The HPLC method of Li and Fitzloff[10] was used to determine the hydrastine and berberine content in powders, capsules, and tablets.

Sample preparation: Extract one capsule with 15 mL of 90% methanol (containing 1% acetic acid) by sonication for 60 minutes and let stand overnight. Filter the solution and then extract with 15 mL of methanol (containing 1% acetic acid) by sonication for 30 minutes. Filter the solution into a flask and wash the residue with three 15-mL portions of methanol. Combine the extracts, and evaporate to dryness under reduced pressure. Dissolve the residue in 10 mL of methanol for HPLC analysis.

Chromatography

Column: Supelco Discovery C18, 5 μm, 250 × 4.6 mm.

Mobile phase: Solvent A = water (containing 10% acetonitrile and 0.1% trifluoroacetic acid), solvent B = acetonitrile (containing 0.1% trifluoroacetic acid).

Gradient:

Time (minutes)	%A	%B
0	90	10
20	40	60

Flow rate: 1.0 mL/minute

Injection volume: 10 μL

Detection wavelength: 225 nm

Column temperature: 20°C

Validation data:

Linearity: 10 to 200 mcg/mL with a correlation coefficient over 0.999 for berberine and hydrastine.

Accuracy: The average percent recoveries were 98.25 and 104.2 for berberine and hydrastine, respectively.

Precision: Not specified
Selectivity: Peak identification was determined against standards.
Ruggedness: Not specified
Robustness: Not specified
LOD/LOQ: LOD = 0.1 mcg/mL for both compounds; LOQ = 0.4 mcg/mL for both compounds.

Method 3: The HPLC method of Weber et al.[11] was used to determine berberine, hydrastine, canadine, and palmatine.

Sample preparation: Extract 0.3 to 2 g of powdered roots with 100 mL of acetonitrile–water–phosphoric acid (70:30:0.1 vol/vol/vol). Sonicate the sample at ambient temperature for 5 minutes, shake on wrist-action shaker for 10 minutes, and then centrifuge at 2200 rpm for 5 minutes.

Chromatography

Column: Zorbax Eclipse XDB-C18, 80Å, 3.5 μm, 150 × 4.6 mm with Zorbax Eclipse XDB-C18, 80Å, 5 μm, 12.5 × 4.6 mm guard column.
Mobile phase: Solvent A = buffer solution (30 mM ammonium acetate–14 mM triethylamine, adjusted to pH 4.85 with acetic acid), solvent B = acetonitrile. A/B, 680/320 vol/vol, isocratic.
Flow rate: 1.0 mL/minute
Injection volume: 10 μL
Detection wavelength: 230 nm
Column temperature: 30°C

Validation data:

Linearity: For palmatine, 0.439 to 8.760 mcg/mL with a correlation coefficient of 0.99999; for berberine, 5.220 to 103.560 mcg/mL with a correlation coefficient of 0.99998; for hydrastine, 5.490 to 109.2 mcg/mL with a correlation coefficient of 0.99994; and for canadine, 0.462 to 9.060 mcg/mL with a correlation coefficient of 0.99996.
Accuracy: Palmatine = 92.3% recovery, berberine = 101.5%, canadine = 101.6%, and hydrastine = 101.9%.
Precision: The RSDs for all four alkaloids were less than 1.6%.
Selectivity: Peak identification was determined against standards.
Ruggedness: Less than 5% RSD between two chemists.
Robustness: Not specified
LOD/LOQ: Not specified

Method 4: The HPLC method of Wang et al.[1] was used to determine the hydrastine and berberine content in powders, capsules, and tablets.

Sample preparation: Extract 100 mg of root powder or extract with 35 mL of 50% methanol (containing 2% of concentrated hydrochloric acid) by sonication for 25 minutes and shaking for 15 minutes. Cool to room temperature and dilute to volume using 50% methanol (containing 2% concentrated hydrochloric acid).

Chromatography

Column: Phenomenex Luna Phenylhexyl, 3 μm, 150 × 4.6 mm.

Mobile phase: Acetonitrile–isopropanol–water–phosphoric acid (34:10:56:0.2 vol/vol/vol/vol) with sodium lauryl sulfate added to achieve the final concentration of 5 mM.

Flow rate: 1.2 mL/minute

Injection volume: 10 μL

Detection wavelength: 235 nm

Validation data:

Linearity: For hydrastine, 2 to 1000 mcg/mL with a correlation coefficient of over 0.9996; and for berberine, 2 to 800 mcg/mL with a correlation coefficient of over 0.9992.

Accuracy: The percent recoveries were 98.4 and 102.9 for hydrastine and berberine, respectively.

Precision: 2.1% RSD for hydrastine and 1.48% RSD for berberine.

Selectivity: Peak identification was determined against standards.

Ruggedness: 0.49% between two chemists.

Robustness: Not specified

LOD/LOQ: LOQ = 2 mcg for both compounds.

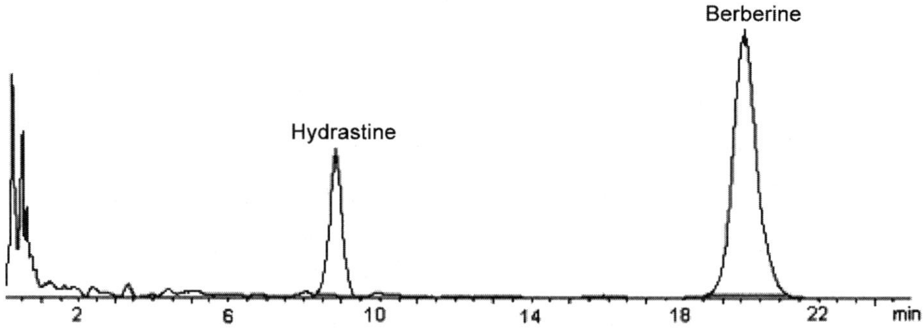

Representative HPLC chromatogram of goldenseal run by method 4.

References

1. Wang M, Zhu N, Jin Y, et al. A quantitative HPLC method for the quality assurance of goldenseal products in the U.S. market. ACS symposium series 803: quality management of nutraceuticals. Washington, DC: American Chemical Society; 2002:199–214.
2. Gentry EJ, Jampani HB, Keshavarz-Shokri A, et al. Antitubercular natural products: berberine from the roots of commercial *Hydrastis canadensis* powder. Isolation of inactive 8-oxotetrahydrothalifendine, canadine, hydrastine, and two new quinic acid esters, hycandinic acid esters-1 and -2. *J Nat Prod*. 1998;61(10):1187–93.
3. Galeffi C, Cometa MF, Tomassini L, et al. Canadinic acid. An alkaloid from *Hydrastis canadensis*. *Planta Med*. 1997;63(2):194.
4. Messana I, La Bua R, Galeffi C. The alkaloids of *Hydrastis canadensis* L. (Ranunculaceae). Two new alkaloids: hydrastidine and isohydrastidine. *Gaz Chim Ital*. 1980;110(9–10): 539–43.
5. Gleye J, Ahond A, Stanislas E. Canadaline. New alkaloid from *Hydrastris canadensis. Phytochemistry.* 1974;13(3):675–6.
6. Nijland MM. The presence of chlorogenic acid in Hydrastis. *Pharm Weekbl*. 1959 Dec.26;94:853–4.
7. Hammond EL. The fat acids of *Hydrastis canadensis* Linne. *Pharm Arch*. 1942;13:17–28.
8. Da Silva AP, Rocha RS, Cristina ML, et al. Antioxidants in medicinal plant extracts. A research study of the antioxidant capacity of Crataegus, Hamamelis and Hydrastis. *Phytother Res*. 2000;14(8):612–6.
9. Abourashed EA, Khan IA. High-performance liquid chromatography determination of hydrastine and berberine in dietary supplements containing goldenseal. *J Pharm Sci*. 2001;90:817–22.
10. Li W, Fitzloff JF. A validated high-performance liquid chromatographic method for the analysis of goldenseal. *J Pharm Pharmacol*. 2002;54(3):435–9.
11. Weber HA, Zart MK, Hodges AE, et al. Method validation for determination of alkaloid content in goldenseal root powder. *J AOAC Int*. 2003;86(3):476–83.

GOTU KOLA

Description

Botanical names: *Centella asiatica* (L.) Urban; *Hydrocotyle asiatica*

Common names: Hydrocotyle, India pennywort

Parts of plant used: Leaves, dried aboveground parts

Uses: To improve memory, to improve blood flow throughout the body by strengthening the veins and capillaries, as a wound-healing agent, as a topical application for skin conditions such as ulcers, wounds, and eczema.

Mode of Action

Several clinical trials have evaluted the health benefits of gotu kola.[1] The total triterpenes fraction has been used to treat edema and to increase capillary filtration in venous hypertension,[2] to treat diabetic microangiopathy by improving microcirculation and decreasing capillary permeability,[3] to improve microcirculation in venous hypertension,[4] and to stimulate maturation of the scar by the production of type 1 collagen.[5]

Chemical Markers

The main chemical components in gotu kola are triterpenes including ursane- and oleanane-type triterpene glycosides. The triterpenes include asiaticoside, madecassoside (asiaticoside A), asiaticoside B, scheffoleoside A, madecassic acid, asiatic acid, terminolic acid, and centellasaponins B, C, and D.[6,7] Other identified components include flavonoids (quercetin, kaempferol, 3-glucosylquercetin, 3-glucosylkaempferol, β-sitosterol, daucosterol, vanillic acid, 11-oxohenicosanyl-cyclohexane, dotriacont-8-1-oic acid, carotenoids, and chlorophyll.[8–11] The essential oils of gotu kola aerial parts were analyzed by GC and GC–MS and the major chemical category found was the sesquiterpenoids, with β-caryophyllene, α-humulene, and germacrene-D as the most abundant.[12] As the triterpenes are the major and also the bioactive components in gotu kola, they are used as chemical markers for quality control of this herb. The marker compounds include asiaticoside, madecassoside, asiatic acid, madecassic acid, terminolic acid, and asiaticoside B.

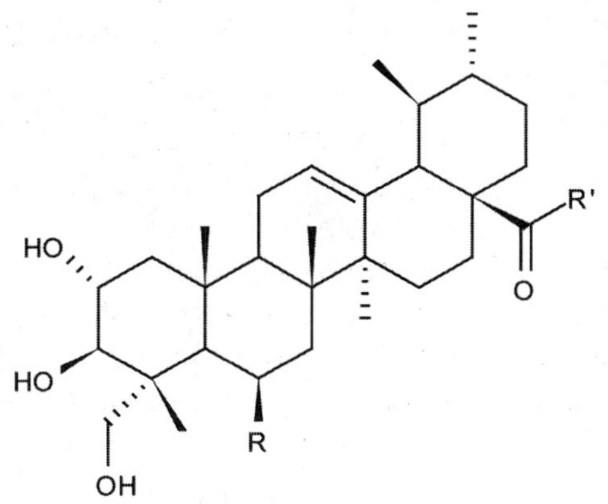

Asiatic acid: R = H, R′ = OH
Madecassic acid: R = OH, R′ = OH
Asiaticoside: R = H, R′ = O-Glu(6-1)-Glu(4-1)-Rham
Madecassoside: R = OH, R′ = O-Glu(6-1)-Glu(4-1)-Rham

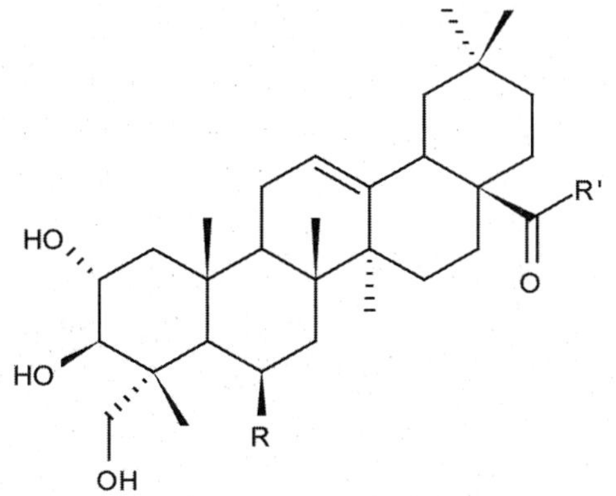

Terminolic acid: R = OH, R′ = OH
Asiaticoside B: R = OH, R′ = O-Glu(6-1)-Glu(4-1)-Rham

Methods of Analysis

Most published analytical methods for total triterpenes in gotu kola use reversed-phase HPLC with gradient elution and low-wavelength detection.[13–17] Most of these methods are not accurate for analysis of triterpenes in gotu kola because they cannot separate madecassic acid from terminolic acid and/or madecassoside from asiaticoside.[13]

Extraction is of key importance for the accurate analysis of total triterpenes. Usually pure methanol, 90% methanol aqueous solution, and 80% methanol aqueous solution are suitable solvents for extraction; organic solvents (acetone, ethyl acetate, chloroform) are not suitable for triterpene glycosides. Triterpenes are not very soluble in water, so the increased level of water in the extraction solvent will decrease the extraction efficacy of triterpenes such as asiatic acid and madecassic acid.

Method 1: Schaneberg et al.[13] were the first to separate totally the six triterpenes of interest: asiaticoside, madecassoside (asiaticoside A), asiaticoside B, madecassic acid, asiatic acid, and terminolic acid.

Sample preparation: Place gotu kola powders (about 500 mg) into a 15-mL screw-cap polypropylene centrifuge tube, and extract three times by sonication for 10 minutes. Centrifuge and transfer the supernates to a 10-mL volumetric flask, and fill to volume with methanol.

Chromatography

Column: Phenomenex Aqua C18, 200 Å, 5 µm, 150 × 4.6 mm guard column (Security Guard C18 cartridge system from Phenomenex).

Mobile phase: Solvent A = water (0.01% trifluoroacetic acid), solvent B = acetonitrile (6% methyl *tert*-butyl ether and 0.01% trifluoroacetic acid), solvent C = acetonitrile (12.0% methyl *tert*-butyl ether and 0.01% trifluoroacetic acid), solvent D = acetonitrile.

Gradient:

Time (minutes)	%A	%B	%C	%D	curve
0	81	19	—	—	0
15	67	33	—	—	10
20	67	0	33	—	6
40	59	—	41	—	10
50	55	—	45	—	—
60	—	—	—	100	—
70	81	19	—	—	—

Flow rate: 1.0 mL/minute

Injection volume: 10 µL

Detection wavelength: 206 nm

Validation data:

Linearity: 5.0 to 850 mcg/mL with a correlation coefficient over 0.995 for all six compounds.

Accuracy: The percent recoveries were from 98.39 to 100.02 for different triterpenes.

Precision: Not specified

Selectivity: Peak identification was determined against standards.

Ruggedness: Not specified

Robustness: Not specified

LOD/LOQ: LOD = 0.010 ng.

Method 2: The unpublished method of Mingfu Wang was used.

Chromatography

Column: Phenomenex Prodigy ODS3, 5 μm, 150 × 3.2 mm.

Mobile phase: Solvent A = water (0.2% phosphoric acid), solvent B = acetonitrile.

Gradient:

Time (minutes)	%A	%B
0	82	18
12	78	22
25	55	45
35	20	80
36	82	18
45	82	18

Flow rate: 1.2 mL/minute

Injection volume: 10 μL

Detection wavelength: 203 nm

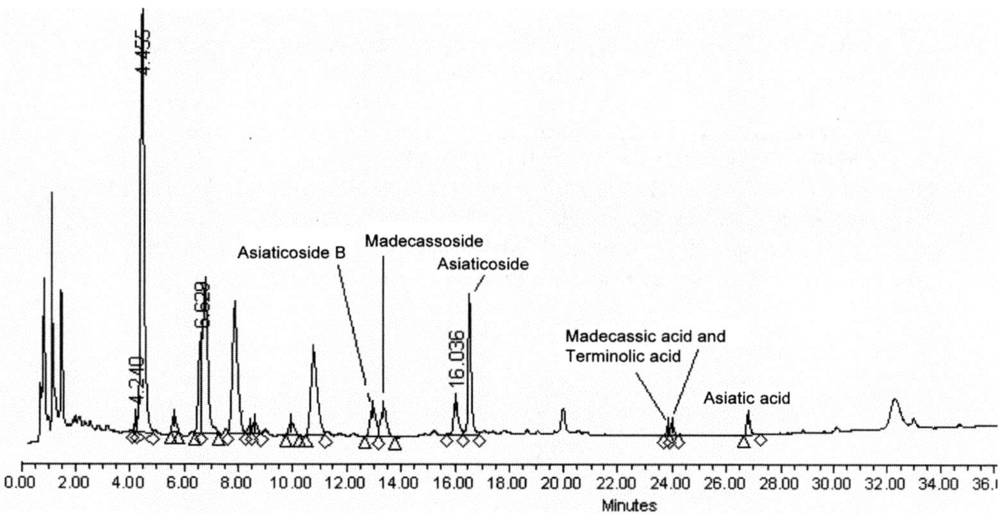

Representative HPLC chromatogram of gotu kola run by method 2.

References

1. Brinkhaus B, Lindner M, Schuppan D, et al. Chemical, pharmacological and clinical profile of the East Asian medical plant *Centella asiatica*. *Phytomedicine*. 2000;7(5):427–48.
2. De Sanctis MT, Belcaro G, Incandela L, et al. Treatment of edema and increased capillary filtration in venous hypertension with total triterpenic fraction of *Centella asiatica*: a clinical, prospective, placebo-controlled, randomized, dose-ranging trial. *Angiology*. 2001;52(Suppl. 2):S55–9.
3. Cesarone MR, Incandela L, De Sanctis MT, et al. Evaluation of treatment of diabetic microangiopathy with total triterpenic fraction of *Centella asiatica*: a clinical prospective randomized trial with a microcirculatory model. *Angiology* 2001;52(Suppl. 2):S49–54.

4. Cesarone MR, Belcaro G, De Sanctis MT, et al. Effects of the total triterpenic fraction of *Centella asiatica* in venous hypertensive microangiopathy: a prospective, placebo-controlled, randomized trial. *Angiology.* 2001;52(Suppl. 2): S15–8.
5. Widgerow AD, Chait LA, Stals R, et al. New innovations in scar management. *Aesthetic Plast Surg.* 2000;24(3):227–34.
6. Matsuda H, Morikawa T, Ueda H, et al. Medicinal foodstuffs. XXVII. Saponin constituents of gotu kola (2): structures of new ursane- and oleanane-type triterpene oligoglycosides, centellasaponins B, C, and D, from *Centella asiatica* cultivated in Sri Lanka. *Chem Pharm Bull.* 2001;49(10):1368–71.
7. Srivastava R, Shukla YN, Kumar S. Chemistry and pharmacology of *Centella asiatica*: a review. *J Med Aromatic Plant Sci.* 1997;19(4):1049–56.
8. He MF, Meng ZM, Wo LQ. Chemical constituents of *Centella asiatica* (L.) Urb. *Zhongguo Yike Daxue Xuebao.* 2000;31(2):91–3.
9. Rao PS, Seshadri TR. Variation in the chemical composition of Indian samples of *Centella asiatica. Curr Sci.* 1969;38(4):77–9.
10. Prum N, Illel B, Raynaud J. Flavonoid glycosides from *Centella asiatica* L. (Umbelliferae). *Pharmazie.* 1983;38(6):423.
11. Srivastava R, Shukla YN. Some chemical constituents from *Centella asiatica. Indian Drugs.* 1996;33(5):233–4.
12. Wong KC, Tan GL. Essential oil of *Centella asiatica* (L.) Urb. *J Essential Oil Res.* 1994;6(3):307–9.
13. Schaneberg BT, Mikell JR, Bedir E, et al. An improved HPLC method for quantitative determination of six triterpenes in *Centella asiatica* extracts and commercial products. *Pharmazie.* 2003;58(6):381–4.
14. Verma RK, Bhartariya KG, Gupta MM, et al. Reverse-phase high-performance liquid chromatography of asiaticoside in *Centella asiatica. Phytochem Anal.* 1999;10(4):191–3.
15. Laugel C, Baillet A, Ferrier D. Improved HPLC determination of the *Centella asiatica* terpenes: analysis in a multiple emulsion, influence of the surfactants on the retention. *J Liq Chromatogr Relat Technol.* 1998;21(9):1333–45.
16. Inamdar PK, Yeole RD, Ghogare AB, et al. Determination of biologically active constituents in *Centella asiatica. J Chromatogr A.* 1996;742(1–2):127–30.
17. Guenther B, Wagner H. Quantitative determination of triterpenes in extracts and phytopreparations of *Centella asiatica* (L.) Urban. *Phytomedicine.* 1996;3(1):59–65.

GRIFFONIA

Description

Botanical name: *Griffonia simplicifolia*

Common names: 5-HTP, 5-Hydroxytryptophan

Parts of plant used: Seeds

Uses: As an antidepressant, to treat serotonin deficiency syndrome, to treat headache, to control weight.

Mode of Action

L-5-Hydroxytryptophan (5-HTP), a serotonin precursor, is the bioactive component in griffonia seeds. Several double-blind placebo-controlled clinical trials have been performed on this compound. 5-HTP was found to treat headache, to work as an antidepressant drug, to reduce body weight, to treat primary fibromyalgia syndrome, and to inhibit panic.[1–7]

Chemical Markers

L-5-Hydroxytryptophan is the main chemical component in griffonia seeds and a recent study found that the content of 5-HTP can reach 20.83% in the fresh material.[8] Indole-3-acetylaspartic acid, 5′-hydroxyindole-3-acetic acid, griffonin, and griffonilide were also detected in griffonia.[9,10] 5-Hydroxytryptamine was found in the pods and, in lower concentration, in the leaves of mature plants. In griffonia seed oil, the fatty acid composition is 18:2 = 60%, 16:0, 18:0, and 18:1 = 9% to 18%, and 20:0 = 3% to 4%. The main sterols are β-sitosterol (60%), stigmasterol (29%), and campesterol (11%).[11] As 5-HTP has been proven to be the bioactive component, it is used as the marker compound for quality control of griffonia seed extract.

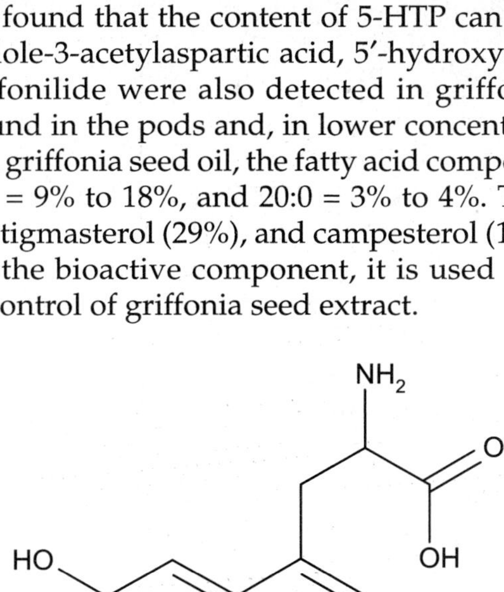

L-5-Hydroxytryptophan

Methods of Analysis

HPLC is the most accepted method for 5-HTP analysis. Various solvents have been used to extract 5-HTP from griffonia seeds; 50% methanol proved to be the most effective solvent.[8]

Method 1: The method of Lemaire and Adosraku[8] was used.

Sample preparation: Transfer 1 g of powdered seed sample to a 100-mL volumetric flask, add 70 mL of 50% methanol, and shake vigorously for 10 minutes. Fill to volume with 50% methanol.

Chromatography

Column: Toso Haas ODS-80TS TSK-GEL9R0, 5 µm, 250 × 4.6 mm.

Mobile phase: Water (5 mM phosphate buffer at pH 4.8)–methanol (97:3) isocratic.

Flow rate: 1.5 mL/minute

Injection volume: 20 µL

Detection wavelength: 275 nm

Validation data: Not available

Method 2: The unpublished method of Mingfu Wang was used.

Sample preparation: Weigh 20 mg of 5-HTP or 100 mg of griffonia seed powder into a 100-mL volumetric flask, add 75 mL of 50% methanol and sonicate for 30 minutes. Cool to room temperature, and fill to volume with 50% methanol.

Chromatography

Column: Phenomenex Luna C18(2), 5 µm, 250 × 4.6 mm.

Mobile phase: Solvent A = water (0.1% trifluoroacetic acid), Solvent B = acetonitrile.

Gradient: 2%B to 16%B in 10 minutes.

Flow rate: 0.8 mL/minute

Injection volume: 10 µL

Detection wavelength: 280 nm

Validation data: Not available

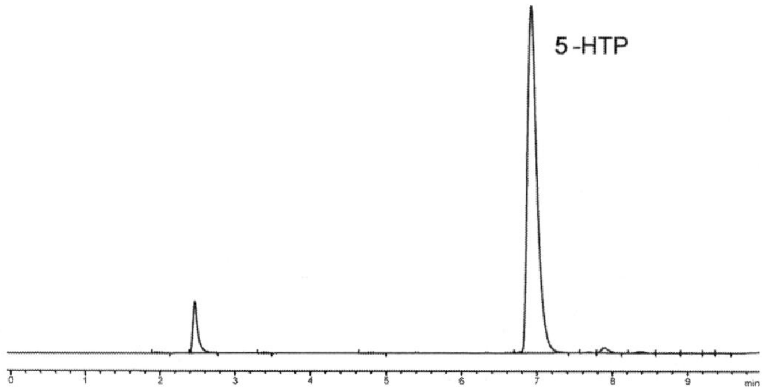

Representative HPLC chromatogram of griffonia seed powder run by method 2.

References

1. Cangiano C, Laviano A, Del Ben M, et al. Effects of oral 5-hydroxytryptophan on energy intake and macronutrient selection in non–insulin dependent diabetic patients. *Int J Obes Relat Metab Disord*. 1998;22(7):648–54.
2. Hirai M. L-5-Hydroxytryptophan as an antidepressant: clinical evaluation and the toxicity of L-5-HTP. *Shinkei Seishin Yakuri*. 1981;3(2):129–34.
3. Schruers K, Van Diest R, Nicolson N, et al. L-5-Hydroxytryptophan-induced increase in salivary cortisol in panic disorder patients and healthy volunteers. *Psychopharmacology*. 2002;161(4):365–9.
4. Schruers K, Van Diest R, Overbeek T, et al. Acute L-5-hydroxytryptophan administration inhibits carbon dioxide–induced panic in panic disorder patients. *J Psychiat Res*. 2002; 113(3):237–43.
5. Ribeiro CA. L-5-Hydroxytryptophan in the prophylaxis of chronic tension-type headache: a double-blind, randomized, placebo-controlled study for the Portuguese Head Society. *Headache*. 2000;40(6):451–6.
6. Cangiano C, Ceci F, Cascino A, et al. Eating behavior and adherence to dietary prescriptions in obese adult subjects treated with 5-hydroxytryptophan. *Am J Clin Nutr*. 1992; 56(5):863–7.
7. Caruso I, Sarzi Puttini P, Cazzola M, et al. Double-blind study of 5-hydroxytryptophan versus placebo in the treatment of primary fibromyalgia syndrome. *J Int Med Res*. 1990; 18(3):201–9.
8. Lemaire PA, Adosraku RK. An HPLC method for the direct assay of the serotonin precursor, 5-hydroxytryptophan, in seeds of *Griffonia simplicifolia*. *Phytochem Anal*. 2002; 13(6):333–7.
9. Dwuma-Badu D, Watson WH, Gopalakrishna EM, et al. Constituents of West African medicinal plants. XVI. Griffonin and griffonilide, novel constituents of *Griffonia simplicifolia*. *Lloydia*. 1976;39(6):385–90.
10. Fellows LE, Bell EA. 5-Hydroxy-L-tryptophan, 5-hydroxytryptamine, and L-tryptophan-5-hydroxylase in *Griffonia simplicifolia*. *Phytochemistry*. 1970;9(11):2389–96.
11. Petkov G, Ramazanov Z. Fatty acids and sterols of Griffonia seeds oil. *Grasas y Aceites*. 2003;54(1):30–1.

GUGGUL

Description

Botanical names: *Commiphora mukul; Balsamodendron mukul; Commiphora wightii*

Common names: Bdellium tree, false myrrh, guggulu

Parts of plant used: Gum resin

Uses: Treatment of hyperlipidemia, reduction of lipid and cholesterol levels

Mode of Action

Several clinical trials have established the activity of guggul[1,2] and guggulsterones were found to be the bioactive components.[3] Guggulsterones were found to be an antagonist of the farnesoid X receptor and an antagonist of the bile acid receptor, to decrease expression of bile acid–activated genes, and to be a farnesoid X receptor antagonist in coactivator association assays. However, guggulsterones act to enhance transcription of the bile salt export pump.[4–6]

Chemical Markers

Guggul resin is a complex mixture of various types of compounds including sterols, diterpenes, triterpenes, lignans, lipids, aliphatic esters, and ferulates.[7–13] The Z-guggulsterone and E-guggulsterone were found to be the bioactive components responsible for the lipid- and cholesterol-lowering activities. Other sterols purified from the gum include guggulsterols I, II, III, IV, V, and VI. The essential oil of guggul gum resin was found to include α-pinene, myrcene, cadinene, geraniol, methylheptanone, and eugenol.[14] E- and Z-Guggulsterones are used as marker compounds for quality control of guggul gum and gum extracts.

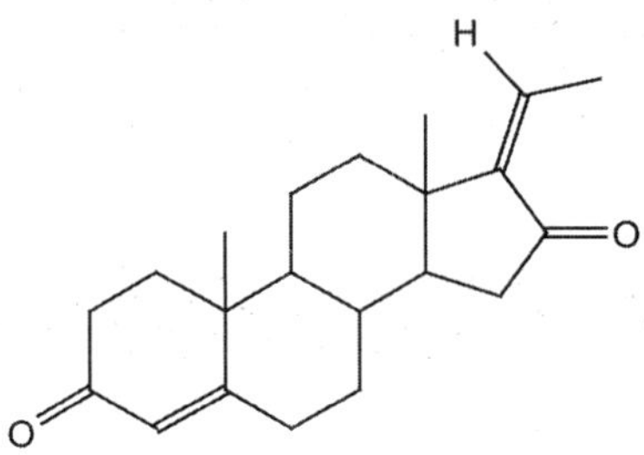

Z-Guggulsterone

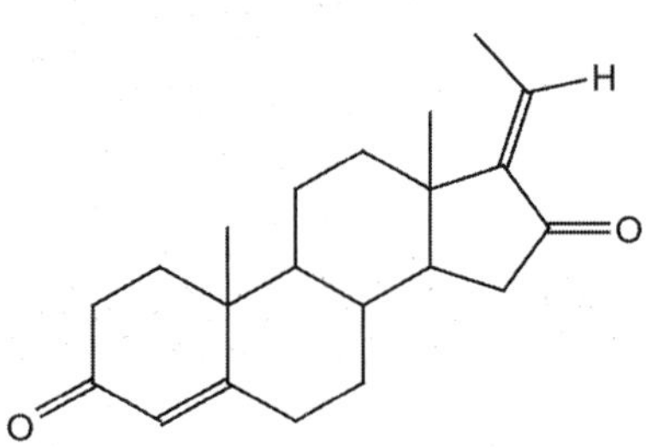

E-Guggulsterone

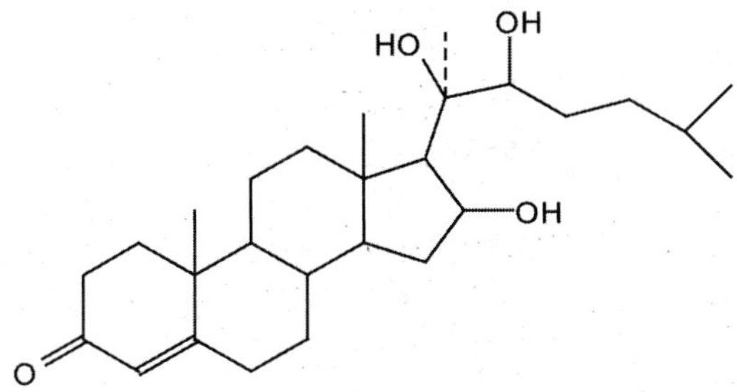

Guggulsterol I

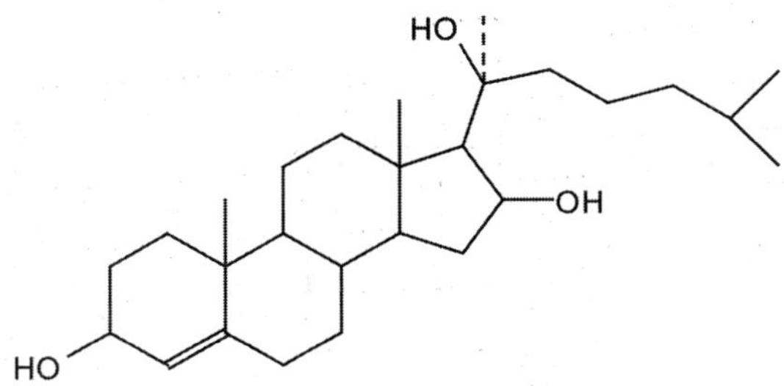

Guggulsterol II

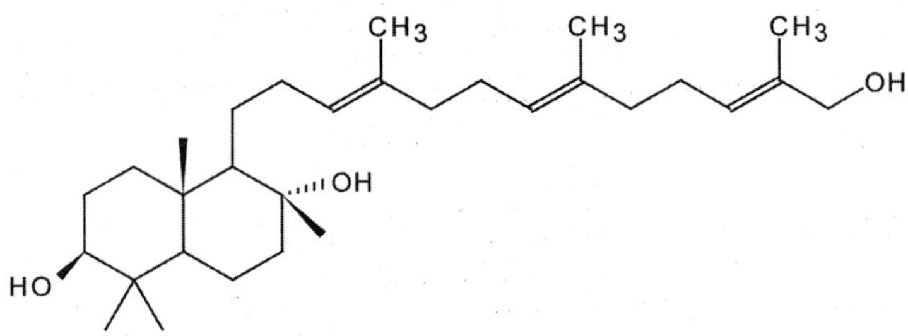

Myrrhanol A

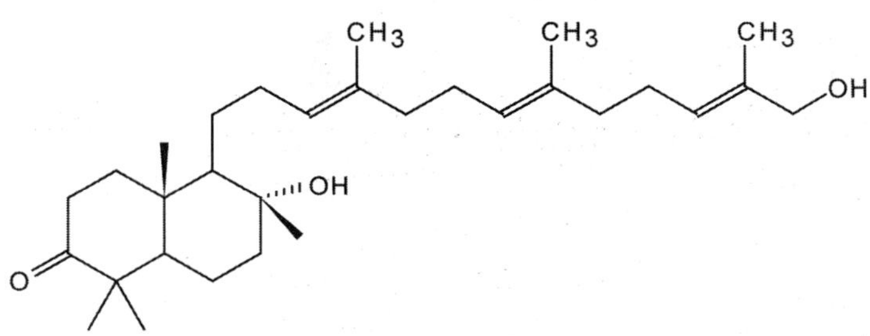

Myrrhanone A

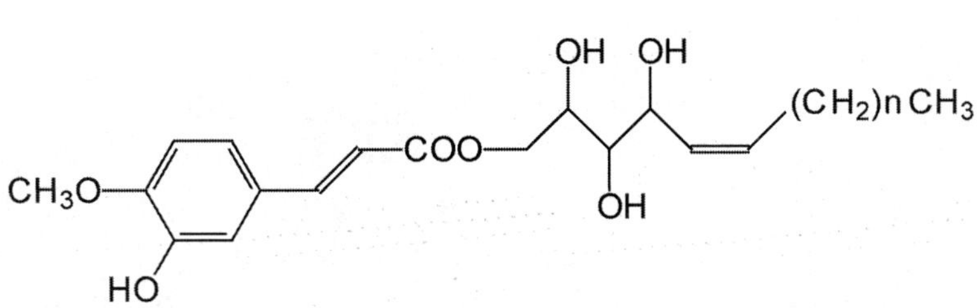

Ferulates: n=16, 17, 18, 19

Methods of Analysis

Several HPLC methods have been developed to determine E- and Z-guggulsterones; an LC–MS method was also reported that could identify the chemical components of guggul.

E- and Z-Guggulsterones can be extracted by organic solvents such as ethyl acetate and methanol. The E- and Z-guggulsterones can also be extracted from a guggul extract with 60% acetonitrile.

Method 1: The method of Mesrob et al.[15] was used.

Sample preparation: Weigh 25 to 30 mg of the resinous extract; dissolve in 2 mL of ethyl acetate, and then dilute to 10 mL with methanol for HPLC analysis.

For commercial tablets, capsules, or powdered extract, grind first, then extract 2 to 3 g three times with 20 mL of ethyl acetate with magnetic stirring for 30 minutes. Dry the ethyl acetate extract. Dissolve 25 to 30 mg of the residue in 2 mL of ethyl acetate and dilute to 10 mL with methanol.

Chromatography

Column: Alltech Adsorbosphere HS-C18, 5 μm, 150 × 4.6 mm.

Mobile phase: Solvent A = water, solvent B = acetonitrile.

Gradient:

Time (minutes)	%A	%B	Curve
0	64	36	—
30	64	36	—
50	55	45	6
56	55	45	—
66	0	100	1
67	64	36	6
76	64	36	—

Flow rate: 1.2 mL/minute

Injection volume: 20 μL

Detection wavelength: 245 nm

Validation data:

Linearity: For Z- and E-guggulsterones, 15 to 85 and 25 to 130 mcg/mL, respectively, with a correlation coefficient over 0.992.

Accuracy: The percent recoveries were from 100 to 103.9 for Z- and E-guggulsterones with two different HPLC systems.

Precision: Not specified

Selectivity: Peak identification was determined against standards.

Ruggedness: Not specified

Robustness: Not specified

LOD/LOQ: Not specified

Method 2: The method of Nagarajan et al.[16] was used.

Sample preparation: Sonicate sample equivalent to 3.0 mg of E- and Z-guggulsterones with acetonitrile in a 50-mL volumetric flask for 30 minutes.

Chromatography

Column: Waters Symmetry C18, 4 μm, 150 × 3.9 mm, with a Sentry C18 guard column, 4 μm, 20 × 3.9 mm.

Mobile phase: Solvent A = water, solvent B = acetonitrile; A:B = 54:46.

Flow rate: 1.0 mL/minute

Injection volume: 20 μL

Column temperature: 25°C

Detection wavelength: 242 nm

Validation data:

Linearity: For both compounds, 0.01 to 0.2 mg/mL with a correlation coefficient over 0.999.

Accuracy: The percent recoveries were 98.7, 99.0, and 97.7 with 50%, 100%, and 150% spiking levels, respectively.

Precision: RSD is less than 2.3%.

Ruggedness: Not specified

Robustness: Not specified

Selectivity: Peak identification was determined against standards.

LOD/LOQ: LOD = 0.005 mg/mL; LOQ = 0.014 mg/mL.

Method 3: The Chromadex method was used; it can be found at www.chromadex.com.

Sample preparation: Extract about 350 mg of guggul extract with 50 mL of 60% acetonitrile in a 100-mL volumetric flask. First shake the sample for 15 minutes and then sonicate for 15 minutes. Cool to room temperature and fill to volume with 60% acetonitrile.

Chromatography

Column: Phenomenex Luna C18(2), 5 μm, 150 × 4.6 mm.

Mobile phase: Solvent A = water–acetonitrile–85% phosphoric acid (50:50:0.1), solvent B = water–acetonitrile–85% phosphoric acid (25:75:0.1).

Gradient:

Time (minutes)	%A	%B
0	100	0
20	0	100

Flow rate: 1.5 mL/minute
Injection volume: 20 μL
Detection wavelength: 241 nm
Column temperature: 25°C

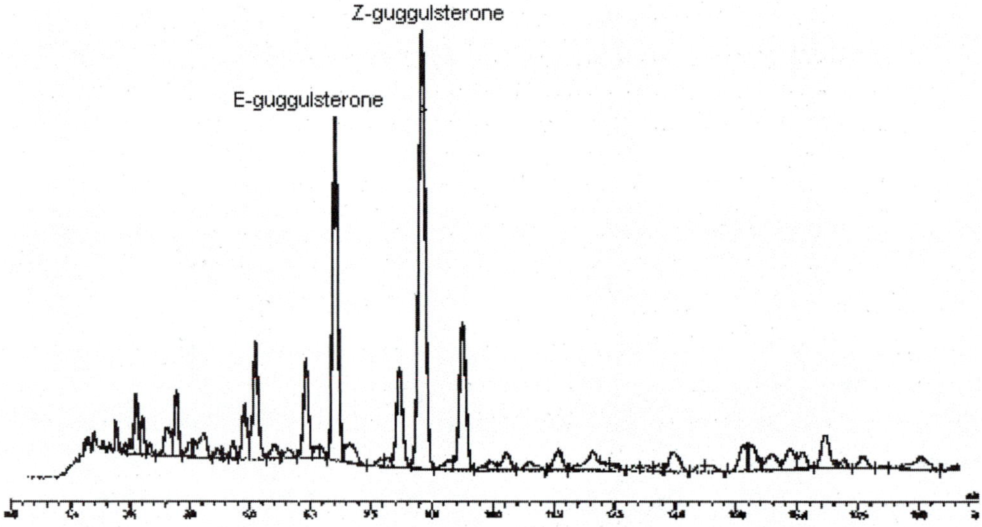

Representative HPLC chromatogram of guggul run by method 3.

References

1. Thompson CJS, Ernst E. Herbs for serum cholesterol reduction: a systematic view. *J Family Pract*. 2003;52(6):468–78.
2. Malhotra SC, Ahuja MM, Sundaram KR. Long-term clinical studies on the hypolipidaemic effect of *Commiphora mukul* (Guggulu) and clofibrate. *Indian J Med Res*. 1977;65(3):390–5.
3. Chander R, Khanna AK, Kapoor NK. Lipid-lowering activity of guggulsterone from *Commiphora mukul* in hyperlipemic rats. *Phytother Res*. 1996;10(6):508–11.
4. Cui J, Huang L, Zhao A, et al. Guggulsterone is a farnesoid X receptor antagonist in coactivator association assays but acts to enhance transcription of bile salt export pump. *J Biol Chem*. 2003;278(12):10214–20.
5. Wu J, Xia C, Meier J, et al. The hypolipidemic natural product guggulsterone acts as an antagonist of the bile acid receptor. *Mol Endocrinol*. 2002;16(7):1590–7.
6. Urizar NL, Liverman AB, Dodds DT, et al. A natural product that lowers cholesterol as an antagonist ligand for FXR. *Science*. 2002;296(5573):1703–6.
7. Zhu N, Rafi MM, DiPaola, et al. Bioactive constituents from gum guggul (*Commiphora wightii*). *Phytochemistry*. 2001;56(7):723–7.

8. Kimura I, Yoshikawa M, Kobayashi S, et al. New triterpenes, myrrhanol A and myrrhanone A, from guggul-gum resins, and their potent anti-inflammatory effect on adjuvant-induced air-pouch granuloma of mice. *Bioorg Med Chem Lett*. 2001;11(8):985–9.
9. Sarkhel S, Yadava U, Prakas P, et al. Guggulsterone E, a lipid-lowering agent from *Commiphora mukul*. *Acta Crystallogr, Section E: Structure Reports Online*. 2001;E57(3): o285–6.
10. Bajaj AG, Dev S. Chemistry of ayurvedic crude drugs. V. Guggulu (resin from *Commiphora mukul*). 5. Some new steroidal components and stereochemistry of guggulsterol-I at C-20 and C-22. *Tetrahedron*. 1982;38(19):2949–54.
11. Patil VD, Nayak UR, Dev S. Chemistry of ayurvedic crude drugs. III. Guggulu (resin from *Commiphora mukul*). 3. Long-chain aliphatic tetrols, a new class of naturally occurring lipids. *Tetrahedron*. 1973;29(11):1595–8.
12. Patil VD, Nayak UR, Dev S. Chemistry of ayurvedic crude drugs. II. Guggulu (resin from *Commiphora mukul*). 2. Diterpenoid constituents. *Tetrahedron*. 1973:29(2):341–8.
13. Patil VD, Nayak UR, Dev S. Chemistry of ayurvedic crude drugs. I. Guggulu (resin from *Commiphora mukul*). 1. Steroidal constituents. *Tetrahedron*. 1972;28(2):2341–52.
14. Saxena VK, Sharma RN. Constituents of the essential oil from *Commiphora mukul* gum resin. *J Med Aromatic Plant Sci*. 1998;20(1):55–6.
15. Mesrob B, Nesbitt C, Misra R, et al. High-performance liquid chromatographic method for fingerprinting and quantitative determination of E- and Z-guggulsterones in *Commiphora mukul* resin and its products. *J Chromatogr B Biomed Sci Appl*. 1998;720(1–2): 189–96.
16. Nagarajan M, Waszkuc TW, Sun J. Simultaneous determination of E- and Z-guggulsterones in dietary supplements containing *Commiphora mukul* extract (guggulipid) by liquid chromatography. *J AOAC Int*. 2001;84(1):24–8.

HOPS

Description

Botanical name: *Humulus lupulus*

Parts of plant used: Dried pistillate inflorescence/strobiles

Uses: As a sedative to treat restlessness and insomnia.

Mode of Action

Hops, a well-known flavoring and preservative ingredient in the brewing of beer, is also bioactive. Clinical trials have proven the sedative effect of the hops extract. Although there were reports about the sedative-hypnotic activity of one component of hops oil (2-methyl-3-buten-2-ol, which is formed through the degradation of bitter acids, that is, α-and β-acids), the components responsible for the activity of hops are still unknown.[1–3]

Chemical Markers

Hops contains numerous phytochemicals. The bitter acids, which are responsible for the characteristic bitterness of hops, are the main component. Their concentration usually is greater than 15% and can reach 30%. Two types of bitter acids are present in the plants: α-acids (humulone, cohumulone, adhumulone) and β-acids (colupulone, lupulone, adluputone).[4] During beer brewing, the α-acids are converted to iso-α-acids, which impart to beer its typical bitter taste. Hops is known to contain flavonoids such as rutin and quercitrin, isoprenylated flavonoids such as 8-prenylnaringenin, isoxanthohumol, and xanthohumol.[5,6] Several flavonoids were identified in hops by MS and LC–MS and proanthocyanidins also were found in hops.[7–9] Hops also contains 0.3% to 1% oil, which is a complex mixture of hydrocarbons, esters, aldehydes, ketones, and alcohols.[10] The bitter acids (six major ones) are used as marker compounds for quality control of hops extract in the U.S. market.

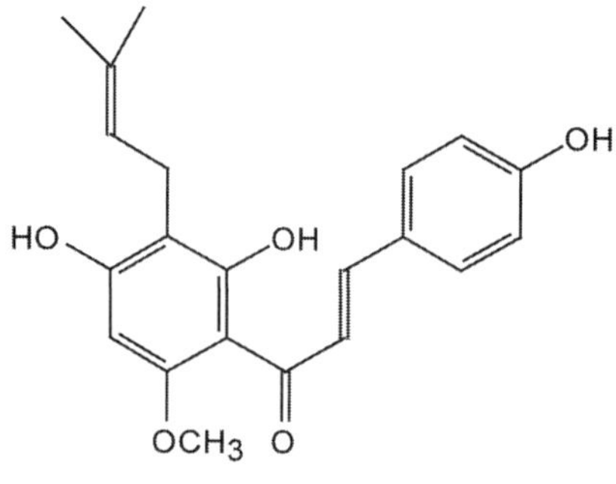

Xanthohumol

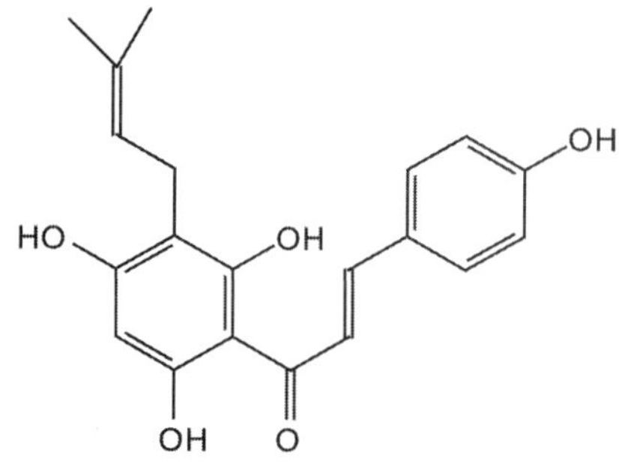

Desmethylxanthohumol

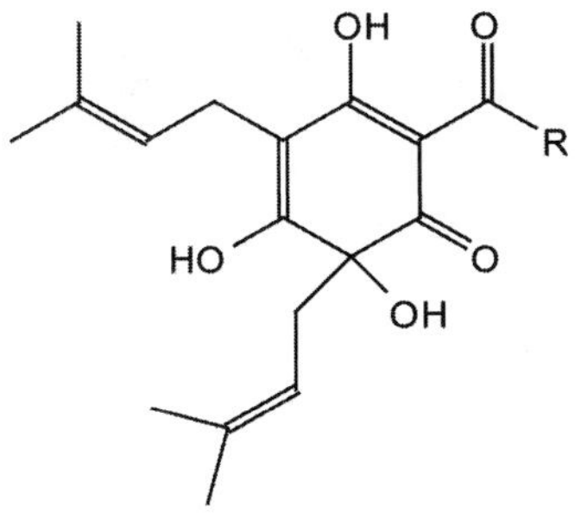

Cohumulone: R = $CH(CH_3)_2$
Humulone: R = $CH_2CH(CH_3)_2$
Adlumulone: R = $CH(CH_3)CH_2CH_3$

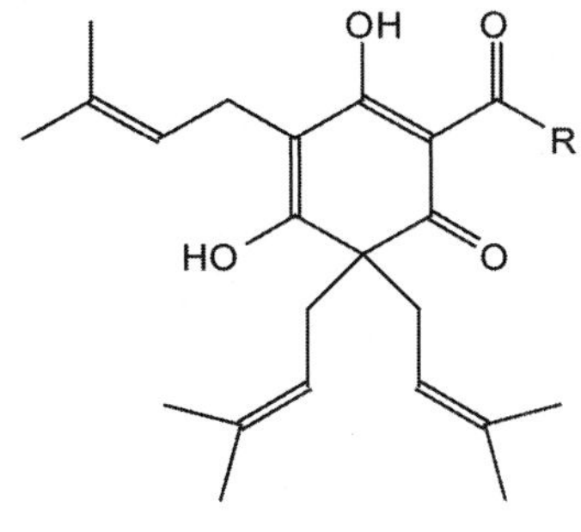

Colupulone: R = $CH(CH_3)_2$
Lupulone: R = $CH_2CH(CH_3)_2$
Adlupulone: R = $CH(CH_3)CH_2CH_3$

Methods of Analysis

Hops is an important flavoring agent for beers, and various methods have been used for the analysis of hops, especially the bitter acids. Due to the instability of the bitter acids of hops, GC is not a good method. HPLC and capillary electrophoresis (micellar electrokinetic chromatography and microemulsion electrokinetic chromatography) are suitable for bitter acids analysis.

Method 1: The method of Hermans-Lokkerbol and Verpoorte[11] was used.

Sample preparation: Dissolve the sample in methanol, and centrifuge before injection.

Chromatography

Column: Phenomenex Hypersil C18, 5 μm, 250 × 4.6 mm.

Mobile phase: 0.05 M Triethanolamine in water–methanol (35:65 vol/vol), pH adjusted to 6.86 with phosphoric acid.

Flow rate: 1.75 mL/minute

Injection volume: Not mentioned

Detection wavelength: 325 nm for α-acids and 358 nm for β-acids.

Validation data:

LOD/LOQ: 25, 20, and 24 ng for humulone, cohumulone, and adhumulone, respectively, and 46, 33, and 41 ng for corresponding lupulones.

Method 2: The method of De Keukeleire et al.[12] was used.

Sample preparation: Grind a hops sample (250 mg to 1 g), suspend in 10 mL of methanol containing 0.01% formic acid, and stir for 1 hour.

Chromatography

Column: Varian Omnisphere C18, 250 × 4.6 mm.

Mobile phase: Solvent A = water (0.025% formic acid), solvent B = methanol (0.025% formic acid).

Gradient:

Time (minutes)	%A	%B
0	55	45
3	55	45
32	5	95
37	5	95
45	55	45
47	55	45

Flow rate: 1 mL/minute

Injection volume: 20 μL

Detection wavelength: 314 nm for α- and β-acids and 370 nm for xanthohumol and desmethylxanthohumol.

Column temperature: 35°C

Method 3: The unpublished method of Mingfu Wang was used.

Sample preparation: Sonicate about 200 mg of hops extract in 35 mL of methanol for 20 minutes, cool to room temperature, and fill to 50 mL.

Chromatography

Column: Phenomenex Luna Phenylhexyl, 3 μm, 150 × 4.6 mm, with guard cartridge.

Mobile phase: Solvent A = water (0.1% formic acid), solvent B = acetonitrile (0.1% formic acid).

Gradient:

Time (minutes)	%A	%B
0	40	60
4	40	60
15	25	75
25	10	90

Flow rate: 1.0 mL/minute

Detection wavelength: 330 nm

Injection volume: 10 μL

Column temperature: Ambient

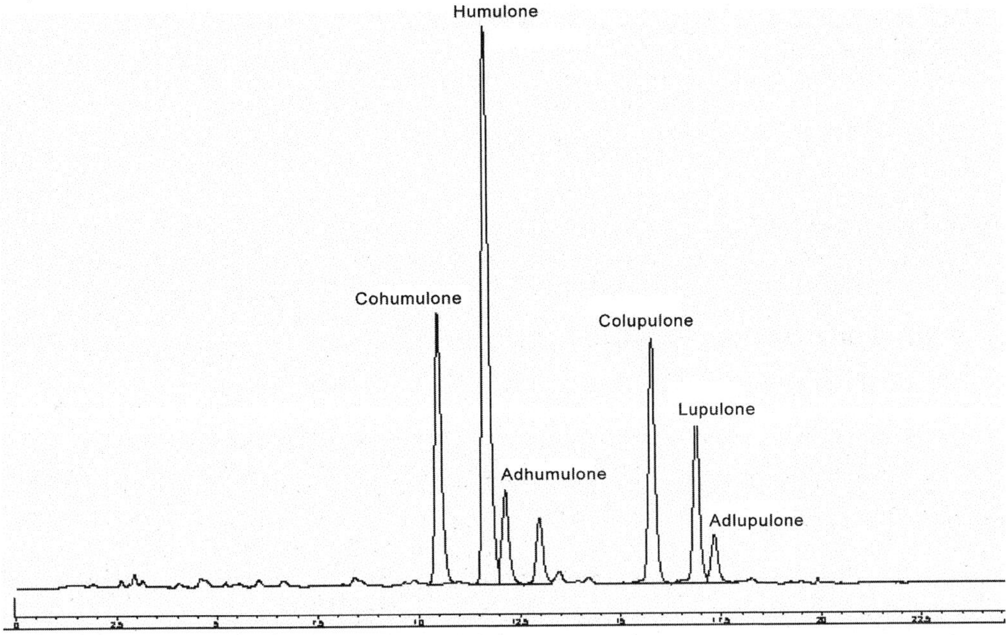

Representative HPLC chromatogram of hops run by method 3.

References

1. Schmitz M, Jackel M. Comparative study for assessing quality of life of patients with exogenous sleep disorders (temporary sleep onset and sleep interruption disorders) treated with a hops-valerian preparation and a benzodiazepine drug. *Wien Med Wochenschr.* 1998;148(13):291–8.
2. Wohlfart R, Hansel R, Schmidt H. The sedative-hypnotic action of hops. 4. Pharmacology of the hop substance 2-methyl-3-buten-2-ol. *Planta Med.* 1983;48(2):120–3.
3. Wohlfart R, Wurm G, Hansel R, et al. Detection of sedative-hypnotic active ingredients in hops. 5. Degradation of bitter acids to 2-methyl-3-buten-2-ol, a hop constituent with sedative-hypnotic activity. *Arch Pharm.* 1983;316(2):132–7.
4. Hu WS, Chu YH. Hop chemistry: recent advances. *Huaxue.* 2002;60(4):A87–106.
5. Stevens JF, Taylor AW, Nickerson GB, et al. Prenylflavonoid variation in *Humulus lupulus*: distribution and taxonomic significance of xanthogalenol and 4′-O-methylxanthohumol. *Phytochemistry.* 2000;53(7):759–75.
6. Stevens JF, Taylor AW, Clawson JE, et al. Fate of xanthohumol and related prenylflavonoids from hops to beer. *J Agric Food Chem.* 1999;47(6):2421–8.
7. Saegesser M, Meinzer M. HPLC-ion spray-tandem mass spectrometry of flavonol glycosides in hops. *J Am Soc Brew Chem.* 1996;54(3):129–34.
8. Stevens JF, Miranda CL, Wolthers KR, et al. Identification and in vitro biological activities of hop proanthocyanidins: inhibition of nNOS activity and scavenging of reactive nitrogen species. *J Agric Food Chem.* 2002;50:3435–43.
9. Walker JR. Phytochemical studies on New Zealand hops. II. Phenolic constituents (or "tannins"). *NZ J Sci.* 1968;11(1):63–71.
10. Walker JR. Phytochemical studies on New Zealand hops. I. Comparison of essential oils by gas-liquid chromatography. *NZ J Sci.* 1967;10(2):476–80.
11. Hermans-Lokkerbol AC, Verpoorte R. Development and validation of a high-performance liquid chromatography system for the analysis of hop bitter acids. *J Chromatogr A.* 1994;669(1–2):65–73.
12. De Keukeleire J, Ooms G, Heyerick A, et al. Formation and accumulation of α-acids, β-acids, desmethylxanthohumol, and xanthohumol during flowering of hops (*Humulus lupulus* L.). *J Agric Food Chem.* 2003;51(15):4436–41.

KAVA

Description

Botanical name: *Piper methysticum* G. Forst.

Common names: Kava kava, kava pepper

Parts of plant used: Roots

Uses: Treatment of sleep disorders, anxiety, stress, and restlessness.

Mode of Action

About 20 clinical trials have proven kava to be effective for treating anxiety and sleep disorders and for improving mental function. The active constituents in kava root consist of a group of structurally related lipophilic lactone derivatives, kavalactones, with an arylethylene-α-pyrone skeleton. Kava extract and individual kavalactones were found to show direct activity on central nervous system receptors and on neurotransmitters. Kavalactones also were found to interact with γ-aminobutyric acid (GABA)–benzodiazepine receptors, to inhibit noradrenaline uptake, and to modulate the voltage-dependent Na^+ and Ca^{2+} channels.[1]

Chemical Markers

Kava roots contain kavalactones as the main chemical components, with the major ones being kavain, 5,5-dihydrokavain, methysticin, dihydromethysticin, yangonin, and desmethoxyyangonin. Currently, 18 kavalactones have been isolated from kava.[2] Other types of compounds identified in kava include alkaloids, chalcones (flavokawains A, B, C), flavanones (pinostrobin, 5,7-dimethoxyflavanone), cinnamic acid derivatives (bornyl ester of 3,4-methylene dioxycinnamic acid, cinnamic acid bornyl ester), long-chain fatty acids and alcohols, and sterols.[2–4] Kavalactones (six main ones) are used as marker compounds for quality control of kava extract in the U.S. market.

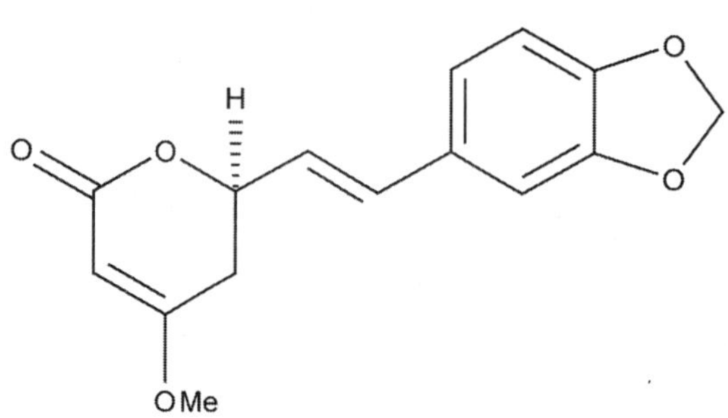

Methysticin

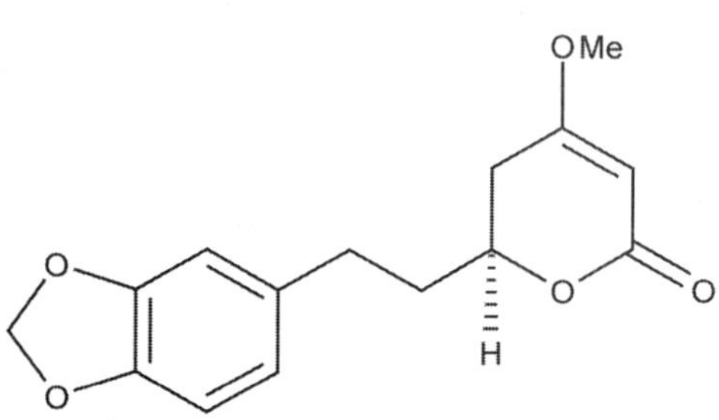

Dihydromethysticin

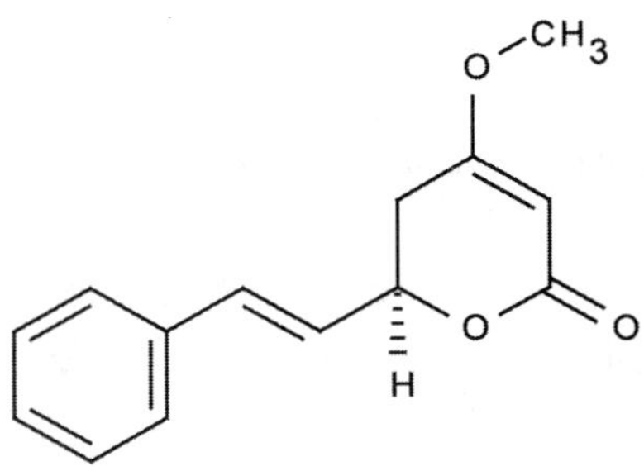

Kavain

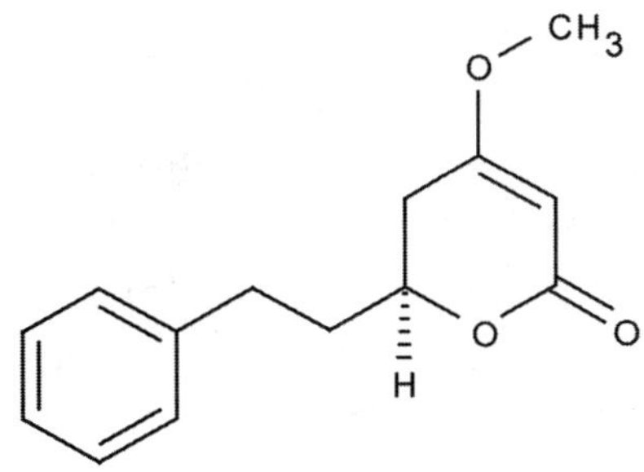

Dihydrokavain

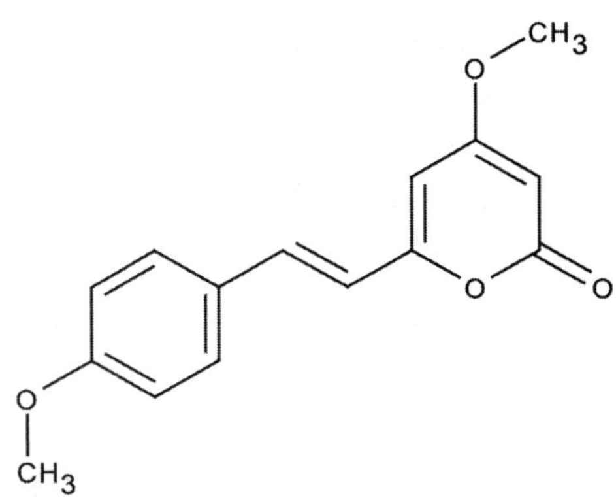

Yangonin

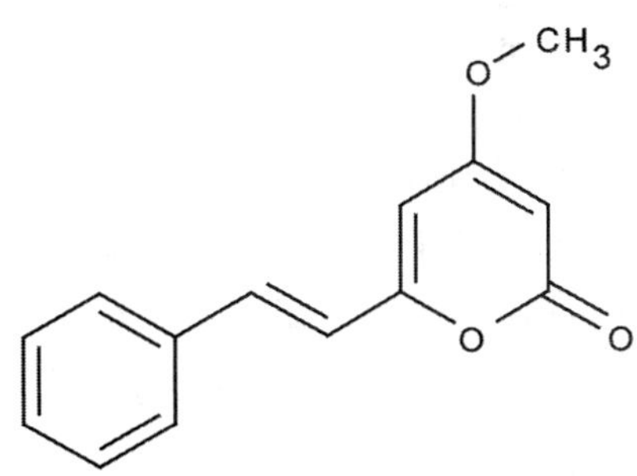

Desmethoxyyangonin

Major kavalactones in kava.

Methods of Analysis

Several methods have been used to determine the total kavalactones in kava including colorimetry, TLC, GC, and HPLC. Currently, the HPLC method is generally used for quality control of kavalactones. The two best HPLC methods for total separation of kavalactones in a short time are as follows.

Method 1: The method found at www.nsfina.org was used.

Sample preparation: For kava herb powders, weigh 750±0.1 mg into a 50-mL volumetric flask, and add 40 mL of methanol–water (70:30). Sonicate for 60 minutes at room temperature. Cool to room temperature and fill to volume with methanol–water (70:30).

For kava paste (50% to 60% kavalactones), weigh about 100 mg into a 50-mL volumetric flask, and add 40 mL of methanol. Sonicate for 10 minutes or until all of the solids are dissolved. Cool to room temperature and fill to volume.

Chromatography

Column: YMCbasic, 5 μm, 250 × 4.6 mm.

Column temperature: 40°C

Mobile phase: 0.1% phosphoric acid–isopropyl alcohol–acetonitrile (64:16:20 vol/vol/vol) isocratic.

Flow rate: 0.6 mL/minute for YMCbasic; 1.0 mL/minute for J'Sphere.

Detection: 220 nm (246 nm alternatively to improve selectivity).

Injection volume: 5 μL

Run time: 30 minutes

Validation data: Not available

Method 2: The method of Schmidt and Molnar[5] was used.

Column: Phenomenex Luna C18, 5 μm, 250 × 4.6 mm.

Mobile phase: Solvent A = water, solvent B = isopropanol.

Gradient: Linear 20%B to 30%B in 16 minutes.

Column temperature: 60°C

Flow rate: 1.4 mL/minute

Detection wavelength: 240 nm

References

1. Bilia AR, Gallori S, Vincieri FF. Kava-kava and anxiety: growing knowledge about the efficacy and safety. *Life Sci.* 2002;70(22):2581–97.
2. Dharmaratne HR, Nanayakkara NP, Khan IA. Kavalactones from *Piper methysticum*, and their ^{13}C NMR spectroscopic analyses. *Phytochemistry.* 2002;59(4):429–33.
3. Wu D, Nair MG, Dewitt DL. Novel compounds from *Piper methysticum* G. Forst. (kava kava) roots and their effect on cyclooxygenase enzyme. *J Agric Food Chem.* 2002;50:701–5.
4. Dragull K, Yoshida WY, Tang CS. Piperidine alkaloids from *Piper methysticum*. *Phytochemistry.* 2003;63(2):193–8.
5. Schmidt AH, Molnar I. Computer-assisted optimization in the development of a high-performance liquid chromatographic method for the analysis of kava pyrones in *Piper methysticum* preparations. *J Chromatogr A.* 2002;948(1–2):51–63.

MELATONIN

Description

Chemical names: N-[2-(5-Methoxy-1H-indole-3-yl)ethyl]acetamide; N-acetyl-5-methoxytryptamine

Molecular weight: 232.28

Chemical formula: $C_{13}H_{16}N_2O_2$

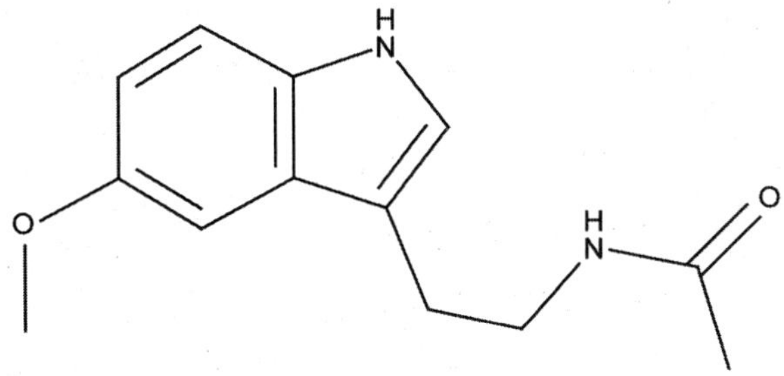

Melatonin

Solubility: Soluble in aqueous solutions, ethanol, and other polar organic solvents.

Other physical/chemical data:

UV max = 223 nm (ε = 27,550), 278 nm (ε = 6300)

Melting point = 116°C to 118°C

Uses: Treatment of insomnia,[1] jet lag,[2] and other sleep disorders. It has also been used to treat depression caused by seasonal affective disorder.[3]

Mode of Action

Melatonin is a naturally occurring hormone that is secreted at night by the pineal gland to help regulate the sleep cycle.

Methods of Analysis

Although many methods have been published for the analysis of melatonin in biological samples, there is little in the literature regarding the analysis of melatonin in dietary supplements. Nevertheless, published methods often can be adapted easily for use with these products. Most methods use reversed-phase HPLC with UV, native fluorescence, derivatization with fluorescence, or electrochemical detection. For the very low levels of melatonin found in biological samples, fluorescence or electrochemical detection is required to obtain the needed sensitivity; however, for dietary supplements, which generally contain between 1 and 20 mg of melatonin per dosage unit, UV detection is sufficiently sensitive. Surprisingly, no method has been published on the analysis of melatonin dietary supplements using HPLC with UV detection.

Melatonin can be extracted from the sample matrix with acidic aqueous buffer, methanol, or other polar organic solvents. It is light sensitive; therefore solutions should be protected from light.

Method 1: Xie et al.[4] used HPLC with electrochemical (EC) detection for the quantitation of melatonin in tablets and capsules. The results were confirmed by MS detection.

Sample preparation: Extract melatonin from tablet and capsule samples with a solution of 20% acetonitrile in 0.1 M perchloric acid using sonication. Filter, and dilute with water to a concentration of between 0.1 and 1 mcg/mL. Inject and analyze by HPLC.

Chromatography

Column: BAS Unijet C18, 5 µm, 150 × 1 mm.

Mobile phase: 20% Acetonitrile–80% buffer [15 mM sodium perchlorate, 40.6 mM sodium citrate, 2.15 mM sodium octylsulfonate, 10 mM diethylamine hydrochloride, and 27 mM disodium edetate (EDTA)].

Flow rate: 100 µL/minute

Column temperature: 35°C

Injection volume: 5 µL

Detection: Electrochemical with a glassy carbon working electrode (3 mm) at an applied voltage of +850 mV versus Ag/AgCl.

Validation data:

Linearity: 0.1 to 1 ng on column (r = 0.9999).

Accuracy: Not specified

Precision: Not specified

Selectivity: Not specified

Ruggedness: Not specified

Robustness: Not specified

LOD/LOQ: LOD = 3 pg on column

Method 2: Cartoni et al.[5] used capillary electrophoresis (CE) with UV detection for the quantitation of melatonin in pharmaceutical tablets.

Sample preparation: Dissolve the tablets in water, filter, and add tryptophan internal standard. Inject this solution on the CE system.

Chromatography

Column: Silica capillary, 44 cm (37 cm to detector) × 50 µm ID, coated with polysiloxane-bonded phase.

Running buffer: 30 mM tetraborate, pH 9.2.

Voltage: 20 kV (44 µA current).

Temperature: 25°C

Injection: Pressure, 10,340 Pa for 0.5 second

Detection: UV at 215 nm

Validation data:

Linearity: 0.01 to 0.10 mg/mL ($r^2 = 0.9983$).

Accuracy: 95.3% to 107% recovery of spiked samples.

Precision: Not specified

Selectivity: Not specified

Ruggedness: Not specified

Robustness: Not specified

LOD/LOQ: LOD = 0.002 mg/mL.

References

1. Zhdanova IV, Wurtman RJ, Lynch HJ, et al. Sleep-inducing effects of low doses of melatonin ingested in the evening. *Clin Pharmacol Ther.* 1995;57:552–8.
2. Petrie K, Dawson AG, Thompson L, Brook R. A double-blind trial of melatonin as a treatment in international cabin crew. *Biol Psychiatry.* 1993;33:526–30.
3. Webb SM, Puig-Domingo M. Role of melatonin in health and disease. *Endocrinology.* 1995;42:221–34.
4. Xie F, Wong P, Yoshioka K, et al. Determination of melatonin in commercially available products by LCEC and LC/MS/MS. *J Liq Chromatogr Relat Technol.* 1998;21:1273–82.
5. Cartoni GP, Coccioli F, Jasionowska R, et al. Rapid analysis of melatonin in pharmaceutical tablets by capillary electrophoresis with UV detection. *Chromatographia.* 2000;52:603.

MILK THISTLE

Description

Botanical name: *Silybum marianum* (L.) Gaertn.

Common name: Mary's thistle

Parts of plant used: Seeds

Uses: As an antihepatotoxic drug to treat alcoholic liver disease and drug-induced liver disease.

Mode of Action

Various clinical trials have been performed on milk thistle that have demonstrated positive effects for indications such as cirrhosis and alcoholic liver diseases, hepatitis, and psychotropic drug–induced liver damage. Silymarin-type flavonolignans are the bioactive components, and they showed antioxidative, antifibrotic, anti-inflammatory, and antilipid activity as well as peroxidative, immunomodulating, and liver-regenerating effects. Silymarin can be used successfully in therapy to promote faster regeneration of diseased liver, and silybinin was found to stimulate the activity of the DNA-dependent RNA-polymerase I, thus increasing the rate of synthesis of all cellular proteins. The increase of protein synthesis offers a good explanation for the liver-regenerating power of milk thistle.[1–4]

Chemical Markers

Milk thistle seed contains a group of compounds that includes flavonolignans, flavonoids, sterols, and fatty acids.[5,6] Silymarins are the bioactive components in milk thistle, and generally the milk thistle extract is expressed as silymarin percentage. Silymarins correspond to a group of flavonolignans, and the major ones are silybin A, silybin B, isosilybin A, isosilybin B, silychristin, and silydianin. Because of the complexities of these structures, the stereochemistry of these compounds, especially the stereochemistry of silybin A and B, and isosilybin A and B was resolved only recently.[7,8] Silymarins are used as marker compounds for quality control of milk thistle extract in the U.S. market.

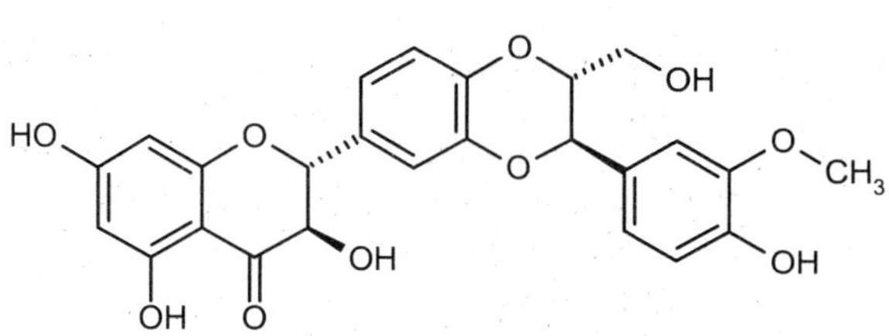

Silybin A

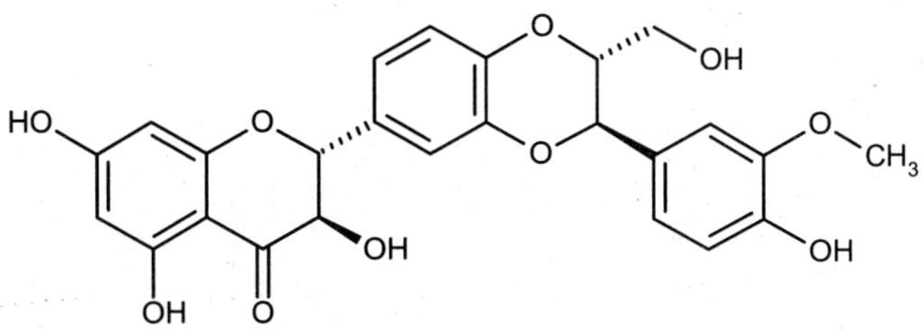

Silybin B

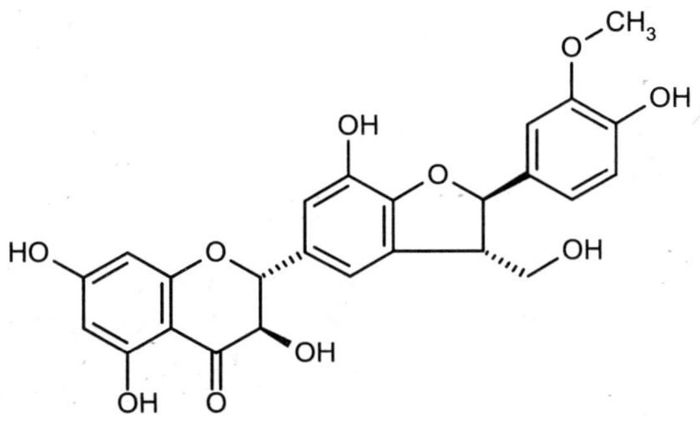

Silychristin

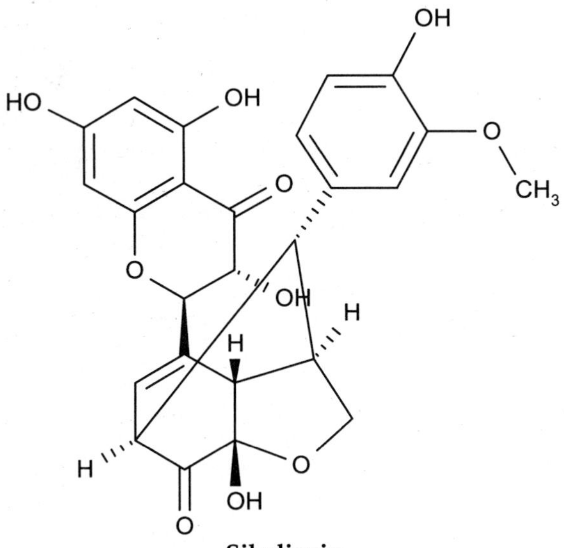

Silydianin

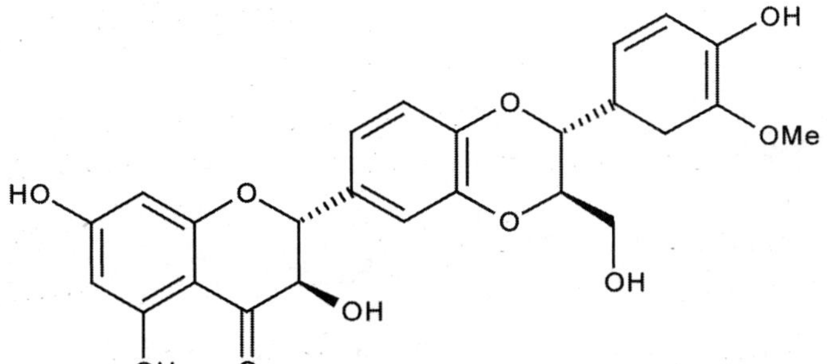

Isosilybin A

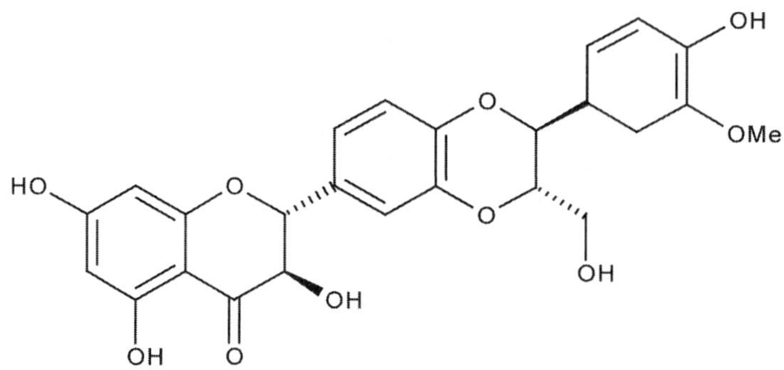

Isosilybin B

Methods of Analysis

The silymarin content in milk thistle has been analyzed by various methods including TLC, HPLC, UV-visible spectrophotometry, and capillary electrophoresis.[9–11] Currently, UV-visible spectrophotometric and HPLC methods are the most accepted for quality control of milk thistle extract. Although many HPLC methods have been published, few methods can separate silybin A from silybin B and isosilybin A from isosilybin B.

Method 1: The method at www.chromadex.com was used. This method can be used to analyze seven compounds including silychristin, silydianin, silybin A, silybin B, isosilybin A, isosilybin B, and taxifolin.

Sample preparation: Weigh 500 mg of milk thistle extract into a 100-mL volumetric flask, add 25 mL of acetonitrile, sonicate for 15 minutes, cool to room temperature, and dilute to volume. Pipette 10 mL of this solution into a 50-mL volumetric flask, and dilute to volume with acetonitrile.

Chromatography

Column: Phenomenex Luna C18(2), 5 μm, 150 × 4.6 mm.

Mobile phase: Solvent A = methanol–water–phosphoric acid (30:70:0.1 vol/vol/vol), solvent B = methanol–water–phosphoric acid (70:30:0.1 vol/vol/vol).

Gradient: 100%A to 100%B in 30 minutes, then keep at 100%B for 5 minutes.

Flow rate: 1.0 mL/minute

Injection volume: 5 μL

Detection wavelength: 288 nm

Validation data: Not available

Method 2: The method at www.nsfina.org was used.

Sample preparation: For fruits, weigh about 10 g of finely ground milk thistle fruit. Transfer the powder into an extraction thimble within a continuous-extraction apparatus (250-mL round-bottom flask containing about 100 mL of hexane). Extract the powder for 4 hours and discard the extract. Transfer the defatted fruit powder to a continuous-extraction apparatus (250-mL round-bottom flask containing about 90 mL of methanol). Extract the powder for 8 hours, cool down, and transfer to a 100-mL volumetric flask and dilute to volume with methanol. Dilute 1:25 with methanol, and filter a portion into an HPLC vial.

For the extract, accurately weigh (±0.1 mg) about 70 mg of extract into a 100-mL volumetric flask. Add 70 mL of methanol and sonicate for 20 minutes. Cool and dilute to volume with methanol.

Chromatography

Column: YMC-Pack ODS-A C18, 5 µm, 150 × 4.6 mm or Phenomenex Luna C18(2), 5 µm, 150 × 4.6 mm.

Mobile phase: Solvent A = methanol–water–phosphoric acid [Mix 200 mL of methanol with 800 mL of water. Mix 5 mL of phosphoric acid into 995 mL of the methanol–water (20:80)], solvent B = methanol–water–phosphoric acid [Mix 800 mL of methanol with 200 mL of water. Mix 5 mL of phosphoric acid into 995 mL of the methanol–water (80:20)].

Gradient:

Time (minutes)	%A	%B
0	85	15
5	85	15
20	55	45
40	55	45
41	85	15
55	85	15

Flow rate: 1.0 mL/minute

Injection volume: 10 µL

Column temperature: 40°C

Detection wavelength: 288 nm

Validation data: Not available, but this method is known to be a validated method.

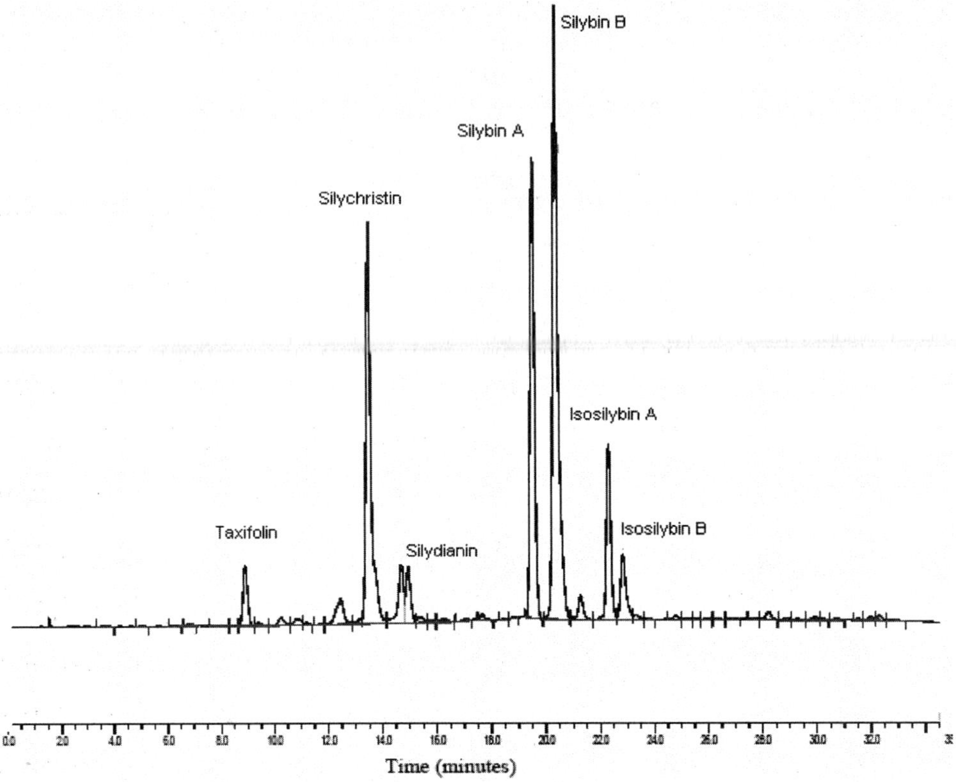

Representative HPLC chromatogram of milk thistle extract run by method 1.

References

1. Saller R, Meier R, Brignoli R. The use of silymarin in the treatment of liver diseases. *Drugs*. 2001;61(14):2035–63.
2. Sonnenbichler J, Sonnenbichler I, Scalera F. Influence of the flavonolignan silybinin of milk thistle on hepatocytes and kidney cells. In: Lawson L, Bauer R, eds. *ACS symposium series 691: phytomedicines of Europe*. Washington, DC: American Chemical Society; 1998:263–77.
3. Luper S. A review of plants used in the treatment of liver disease: part 1. *Altern Med Rev.* 1998;3(6):410–21.
4. Leng-Peschlow E. Properties and medical use of flavonolignans (silymarin) from *Silybum marianum*. *Phytother Res.* 1996;10(Suppl. 1):S25–6.
5. Khafagy SM, Abdel Salam NA, Abdel HR, et al. Constituents of *Silybum marianum* (L.) Gaertn. (Compositae). *Scientia Pharmaceutica*. 1981;49(2):157–61.
6. Yin Q, Wang S, Nan J, et al. Analysis of fatty acids in *Silybum marianum* oil by GC/MS. *Yanbian Daxue Xuebao, Ziran Kexueban*. 1998;24(4):26–8.
7. Lee DY, Liu Y. Molecular structure and stereochemistry of silybin A, silybin B, isosilybin A, and isosilybin B, isolated from *Silybum marianum* (milk thistle). *J Nat Prod.* 2003;66(9):1171–4.
8. Kim NC, Graf TN, Sparacino CM, et al. Complete isolation and characterization of silybins and isosilybins from milk thistle (*Silybum marianum*). *Org Biomol Chem.* 2003; 1(10):1684–9.
9. Kvasnicka F, Biba B, Sevcik R, et al. Analysis of the active components of silymarin. *J Chromatogr A*. 2003;990(1–2):239–45.

10. Bilia AR, Bergonzi MC, Gallori S, et al. Stability of the constituents of calendula, milk thistle and passionflower tinctures by LC–DAD and LC–MS. *J Pharm Biomed Anal.* 2002;30(3):613–24.
11. Quaglia MG, Bossu E, Donati E, et al. Determination of silymarine in the extract from the dried *Silybum marianum* fruits by high-performance liquid chromatography and capillary electrophoresis. *J Pharm Biomed Anal.* 1999;19(3–4):435–42.

OLIVE LEAF

Description

Botanical name: *Olea europaea* L.

Parts of plant used: Leaves

Uses: Treatment and prevention of hypertension; as an antioxidant.

Mode of Action

Very few clinical trials have been performed to validate the use of olive leaf extracts. Olive leaf extracts have shown a blood pressure–lowering effect, hypoglycemic activity, and vasodilator effects, but only in in vitro and in vivo tests. Secoiridoids such as oleuropein found in olive leaf support its hypotensive activity.[1–4] In addition, oleuropein is also a well-known antioxidant.

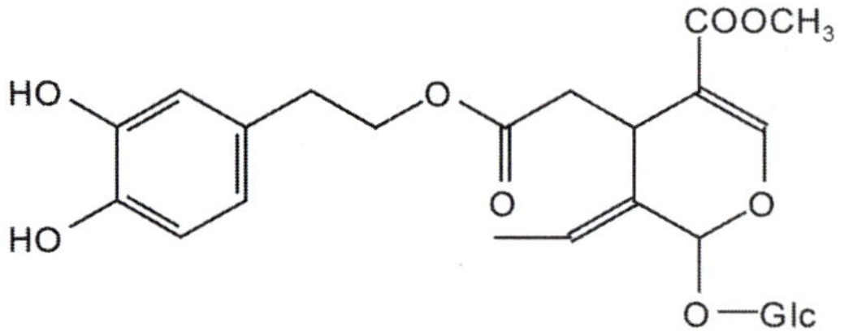

Oleuropein

Chemical Markers

Olive leaf is known to be rich in phenolic compounds. The main phenol identified in olive leaf is oleuropein, a (3,4-dihydroxyphenyl)ethanol ester with β-glucosylated elenolic acid. Other phenolics identified in olive leaf include vanillic acid, caffeic acid, p-coumaric acid, ferulic acid, gallic acid, syringic acid, tyrosol, hydroxytyrosol, apigenin, kaempferol, quercetin, apigenin-7-glucoside, hesperidin, luteolin-7-glucoside, rutin, verbascoside, oleuroside, demethyloleuropein, and ligstroside. The hexane extract of olive leaf was found to contain hydrocarbons, ester waxes, triglycerides, tocopherols, sterols, linear and terpenic alcohols, and terpenic dialcohols. When the volatile compounds were analyzed by GC and GC–MS, mono- and sesquiterpenes were found to be the main volatile components.[2,5–9] Currently, oleuropein is used as a marker compound for quality control of olive leaf extract.

Methods of Analysis

HPLC is a widely used method for analysis of oleuropein; oleuropein is a phenolic compound and can be detected easily by UV.

Method 1: The method of Savournin et al.[2] was used.

Sample preparation: Extract 5 g of dried leaves three times with 30 mL of 60% aqueous methanol, and sonicate for 15 minutes each time. Filter, combine the solutions, and dilute to 100 mL with the same solvent. Dilute the extract solution (1:5) with mobile phase.

Chromatography

Column: Waters Symmetry C18, 5 μm, 250 × 3.9 mm, with a SentryGuard Symmetry C18 guard column, 20 × 3.9 mm.

Mobile phase: Water (adjusted to pH 3 with 0.1 M phosphoric acid)–acetonitrile (adjusted to pH 3 with 0.1 M phosphoric acid).

Gradient: 79:21

Flow rate: 1.0 mL/minute

Injection volume: 20 μL

Detection wavelength: 280 nm

Validation data:

Linearity: Not available

Accuracy: Not specified

Precision: Less than 2% RSD.

Selectivity: Peak identification was determined against standards.

Ruggedness: Not specified

Robustness: Not specified

LOD/LOQ: LOD = 0.4 mcg/mL; LOQ = 0.85 mcg/mL.

Method 2: The method of Del Rio et al.[10] was used.

Sample preparation: Grind the plant material (leaves, stems, roots, cortex, pith), and shake with dimethyl sulfoxide (150 mg of fresh weight per mL) for 1.2 hours.

Chromatography

Column: Spherisorb ODS-2, 5 μm, 250 × 4.0 mm, with a SentryGuard Symmetry C18 guard column, 20 × 3.9 mm.

Mobile phase: Solvent A = water–acetic acid (97.5:2.5), solvent B = acetonitrile.

Gradient: 25%B to 95%B in 50 minutes.
Flow rate: 1.0 mL/minute
Injection volume: 10 μL
Detection wavelength: 280 and 353 nm
Column temperature: 30°C

Validation data: Not specified

Method 3: The method of Ryan et al.[11] was used.

Sample preparation: Blend dried samples (about 0.25 g) with methanol–water (50:50) using an Ultra Turrax blender for 20 seconds, and let the solution stand for 30 minutes. Filter the samples, and extract again using the same procedure, but let stand for 15 minutes. Filter, combine the filtrates, and wash with hexane (5 mL). Use the aqueous phase for HPLC analysis.

Chromatography

Column: Alltech Alltima C18, 5 μm, 150 × 4.6 mm, with a SentryGuard Symmetry C18, 20 × 3.9 mm.
Mobile phase: Solvent A = water–acetic acid (100:1 vol/vol), solvent B = methanol–acetonitrile–acetic acid (95:5:1 vol/vol/vol).
Gradient:

Time (minutes)	%A	%B
0	90	10
30	70	30
40	60	40
50	50	50
55	50	50
60	40	60
65	30	70
70	0	100

Flow rate: 1.0 mL/minute
Injection volume: 10 μL
Detection wavelength: 280 and 353 nm

Validation data: Not specified

Method 4: The unpublished method of Mingfu Wang was used.

Sample preparation: Weigh the appropriate amount of material (120 mg for 15% oleuropein) into a 50-mL volumetric flask. Add approximately 35 mL of 70% methanol, sonicate for 20 minutes, and shake for 20 minutes. Allow the flask to cool to room temperature, and fill to volume with 70% methanol.

Chromatography

HPLC column: Phenomenex Luna C18(2), 5 µm, 250 × 4.6 mm.

Mobile phase: Solvent A = aqueous phosphoric acid (pH 2.5), solvent B = acetonitrile.

Gradient:

Time (minutes)	%A	%B
0	88	12
28	50	50
29	88	12
40	88	12

Column temperature: 30°C

Flow rate: 0.8 mL/minute

Injection volume: 10 µL

Detection wavelength: 254 nm

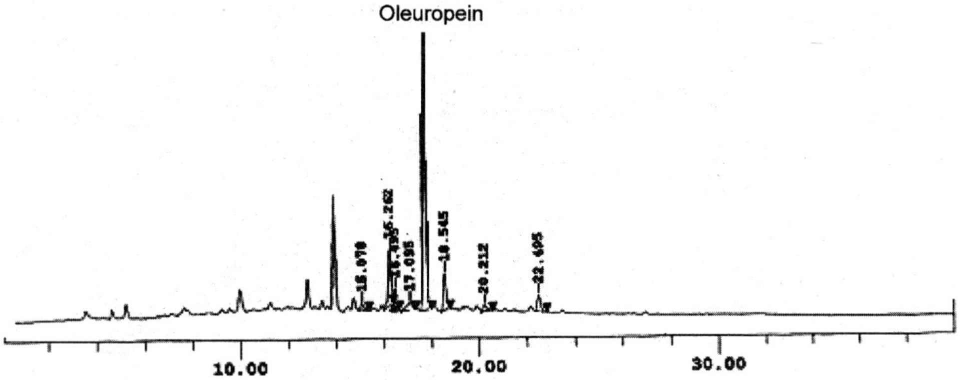

Representative HPLC chromatogram of olive leaf run by method 4.

References

1. Khayyal MT, El-Ghazaly MA, Abdallah DM, et al. Blood pressure–lowering effect of an olive leaf extract (*Olea europaea*) in L-NAME–induced hypertension in rats. *Arzneimittelforschung*. 2002;52(11):797–802.
2. Savournin C, Baghdikian B, Elias R, et al. Rapid high-performance liquid chromatography analysis for the quantitative determination of oleuropein in *Olea europaea* leaves. *J Agric Food Chem*. 2001;49(2):618–21.
3. Gonzalez M, Zarzuelo A, Gamez MJ, et al. Hypoglycemic activity of olive leaf. *Planta Med*. 1992;58(6):513–5.
4. Zarzuelo A, Duarte J, Jimenez J, et al. Vasodilator effect of olive leaf. *Planta Med*. 1991;57(5):417–9.

5. Guinda A, Lanzon A, Rios J, et al. The isolation and quantification of the components from olive leaf: hexane extract. *Grasas y Aceites*. 2002;53(4):419–22.
6. Briante R, Patumi M, Terenziani S, et al. *Olea europaea* L. leaf extract and derivatives: antioxidant properties. *J Agric Food Chem*. 2002;50(17):4934–40.
7. Campeol E, Flamini G, Chericoni S, et al. Volatile compounds from three cultivars of *Olea europaea* from Italy. *J Agric Food Chem*. 2001;49(11):5409–11.
8. De Laurentis N, Stefanizzi L, Milillo MA, et al. Flavonoids from leaves of *Olea europaea* L. cultivars. *Ann Pharm Fr*. 1998;56(6):268–73.
9. Brenes M, Garcia P, Duran MC, et al. Concentration of phenolic compound changes in storage brines of ripe olives. *J Food Sci*. 1992;58:347–50.
10. Del Rio JA, Baidez AG, Botia JM, et al. Enhancement of phenolic compounds in olive plants (*Olea europaea* L.) and their influence on resistance against Phytophthora sp. *Food Chem*. 2003;83(1):75–8.
11. Ryan D, Antolovich M, Herlt T, et al. Identification of phenolic compounds in tissues of the novel olive cultivar Hardy's mammoth. *J Agric Food Chem*. 2002;50(23):6716–24.

PASSIONFLOWER

Description

Botanical name: *Passiflora incarnata* L.

Common names: Apricot vine, maypop, wild passionflower

Parts of plant used: Dried aerial parts

Uses: Treatment of anxiety, nervousness, and minor sleeplessness. Usually used as an infusion or in the form of extracts, mainly combined with other sedative herbs such as hops, kava, and valerian.

Mode of Action

Passiflora incarnata L. is widely used in herbal sedatives. Passionflower is used in combination with hops, valerian, and kava frequently; therefore, clinical studies using this individual herb are not available. Many pharmacological studies confirm the sedative effects of passionflower, and some studies also found anxiolytic effects. Many compounds including maltol, ethyl maltol, indole alkaloids, and flavonoids were found to be responsible, in part, for its activity. However, the mechanism of action is unknown.[1–8]

Chemical Markers

The main chemical components in passionflower are flavone-di-C-glycosides of apigenin and luteolin types including schaftoside, isoschaftoside, isoorientin, orientin, isovitexin, vitexin, saponarin, vicenin-2, and lucenin-2. Passionflower also contains coumarins, maltol, phenolic acids, phytosterols, small amounts of indole alkaloids (harmane, harmine, harmol), and small amounts of essential oil.[9,10] The volatile constituents of *P. incarnata* were investigated by GC, and the main chemicals were identified as hexanal, benzyl alcohol, linalool, 2-phenylethyl alcohol, 2-hydroxybenzoic acid methyl ester, carvone, *trans*-anethole, eugenol, isoeugenol, β-ionone, α-bergamotol, phytol, and two fatty acids (palmitic and oleic).[11] Although the active compounds in passionflower have not been identified, the flavonoids are used as marker compounds for quality control of crude herb and its related preparations.

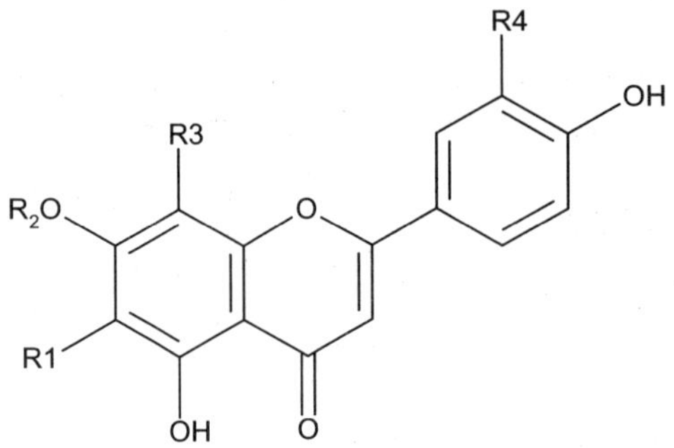

R1	R2	R3	R4	
Glc	H	Glc	H	Vicenin 2
Glc	H	Ara	H	Schaftoside
Ara	H	Glc	H	Isoschaftoside
Glc	H	H	OH	Isoorientin
H	H	Glc	OH	Orientin
Glc	H	H	H	Isovitexin
H	H	Glc	H	Vitexin

Methods of Analysis

Various methods have been developed to analyze the chemicals in passionflower including GC, GC–MS, and GC–FTIR for volatile analysis, HPLC for alkaloids and flavonoid analysis, LC–MS for identifying the flavonoids, capillary electrophoresis for flavonoid analysis, and TLC and colorimetry for determining the total amounts of flavonoids and alkaloids.[12–20]

The flavonoids in passionflower can be extracted easily with methanol, ethanol, or aqueous methanol and ethanol.

Method 1: The method of Bokstaller and Schmidt[19] can be used to identify and quantify the flavonoids vicenin-2, schaftoside, isoorientin, orientin, isovitexin-2-glucoside, vitexin, and isovitexin.

Sample preparation: Prepare samples in 50% ethanol.

Chromatography

Column: Merck LiChrospher 100RP, 5 μm, 250 × 4.0 mm with a guard column LiChrospher 100RP-18, 5 μm, 4 × 4 mm.

Mobile phase: Solvent A = acetonitrile–water (110:690, wt/wt), solvent B = acetonitrile–water (120:180, wt/wt). Both solutions were adjusted to pH 2.8 with phosphoric acid (85%).

Gradient:

Time (minutes)	%A	%B
0	100	0
13	100	0
13.5	0	100
16.5	0	100
17	100	0
25	100	0

Flow rate: 1.2 mL/minute

Injection volume: 10 μL

Detection wavelength: 340 nm

Column temperature: Not controlled

Validation data: Not available

Method 2: The method of Raffaelli et al.[18] can be combined with MS detection to identify 10 flavonoids including vicenin-2, schaftoside, isoschaftoside, isoorientin-2-O-β-glucopyranoside, isoorientin, isovitexin-2-O-β-glucopyranoside, swertisin, orientin, isovitexin, and vitexin.

Sample preparation: Prepare in 50% ethanol.

Chromatography

Column: LiChrospher C18, 250 × 4.6 mm.

Mobile phase: Isocratic condition, water–tetrahydrofuran–isopropanol–acetonitrile (88:8:1.6:2.4); the mobile phase also contained 0.07% formic acid.

Flow rate: 1.0 mL/minute

Injection volume: 10 μL

Detection wavelength: 340 nm

Column temperature: Not controlled

Validation data: Not specified

Method 3: The method of Abourashed et al.[14] was used to analyze six flavonoids — schaftoside, isoschaftoside, isoorientin, orientin, isovitexin, and vitexin — in different species of *Passiflora*.

Sample preparation: Load 2 g of powdered sample onto a stainless steel cartridge, and extract in a Dionex accelerated speed extractor with the following program: solvent = 80% methanol; temperature = 40°C; pressure = 1000 psi; cycle duration = 10 minutes with solvent flush cycle. Repeat three times.

Chromatography

Column: Phenomenex Hypersil ODS, 5 μm, 150 × 4.6 mm with a SecurityGuard cartridge, C18, 4 × 3 mm.

Mobile phase: Solvent A = 0.01% phosphoric acid at pH 3.1, solvent B = acetonitrile–tetrahydrofuran–isopropanol (80:80:20 vol/vol/vol).

Gradient:

Time (minutes)	%A	%B
0	100	0
5	100	0
60	0	100

Between each injection, wash with methanol for 5 minutes, and equilibrate with solvent A for 20 minutes.

Flow rate: 1.0 mL/minute

Injection volume: 10 μL

Detection wavelength: 280 nm

Column temperature: Not controlled

Validation data: Not available

References

1. Krenn L. Passion Flower (*Passiflora incarnata* L.)—a reliable herbal sedative. *Wien Med Wochenschr.* 2002;152(15–16):404–6.
2. Dhawan K, Kumar S, Sharma A. Anxiolytic activity of aerial and underground parts of *Passiflora incarnata. Fitoterapia.* 2001;72(8):922–6.
3. Dhawan K, Kumar S, Sharma A. Anti-anxiety studies on extracts of *Passiflora incarnata* Linneaus. *J Ethnopharmacol.* 2001;78(2–3):165–70.
4. Zanoli P, Avallone R, Baraldi M. Behavioral characterisation of the flavonoids apigenin and chrysin. *Fitoterapia.* 2000;71(Suppl. 1):S117–23.
5. Soulimani R, Younos C, Jarmouni S, et al. Behavioural effects of *Passiflora incarnata* L. and its indole alkaloid and flavonoid derivatives and maltol in the mouse. *J Ethnopharmacol.* 1997;57(1):11–20.
6. Speroni E, Minghetti A. Neuropharmacological activity of extracts from *Passiflora incarnata. Planta Med.* 1988;54(6):488–91.
7. Della LR, Tubaro A, Redaelli C. Evaluation of the activity on the mouse CNS of several plant extracts and a combination of them. *Riv Neurol.* 1981;51(5):297–310.
8. Aoyagi N, Kimura R, Murata T. Studies on *Passiflora incarnata* dry extract. I. Isolation of maltol and pharmacological action of maltol and ethyl maltol. *Chem Pharm Bull.* 1974;22(5):1008–13.
9. Bruneton J. *Pharmacognosy, Phytochemistry, Medicinal Plants.* Paris: Lavoisier Publishing; 1995:284–6.
10. Lutomski J, Segiet-Kujawa E. *Passiflora incarnata* L. Part I. Chemical composition. *Herba Polonica.* 1980;26(1):77–84.
11. Buchbauer G, Jirovetz L. Volatile constituents of the essential oil of *Passiflora incarnata* L. *J Essential Oil Res.* 1992;4(4):329–34.
12. Marchart E, Krenn L, Kopp B. Quantification of the flavonoid glycosides in *Passiflora incarnata* by capillary electrophoresis. *Planta Med.* 2003;69(5):452–6.
13. Bilia AR, Bergonzi MC, Gallori S. Stability of the constituents of calendula, milk thistle and passionflower tinctures by LC–DAD and LC–MS. *J Pharm Biomed Anal.* 2002;30(3):613–24.
14. Abourashed EA, Vanderplank JR, Khan IA. High-speed extraction and HPLC fingerprinting of medicinal plants. I. Application to *Passiflora* flavonoids. *Pharm Biol.* 2002;40(2):81–91.
15. Grice ID, Ferreira LA, Griffiths LR. Identification and simultaneous analysis of harmane, harmine, harmol, isovitexin, and vitexin in *Passiflora incarnata* extracts with a novel HPLC method. *J Liq Chromatogr Relat Technol.* 2001;24(16):2513–23.
16. Voirin B, Sportouch M, Raymond O, et al. Separation of flavone C-glycosides and qualitative analysis of *Passiflora incarnata* L. by capillary zone electrophoresis. *Phytochem Anal.* 2000;11(2):90–8.

17. Petry RD, De Souza KC, Bassani VL, et al. Total flavonoid content determination in aerial parts of *Passiflora alata Dryander* (Maracuja). *Revista Brasileira de Farmacia.* 1998;79(1–2):7–10.
18. Raffaelli A, Moneti G, Mercati V, et al. Mass spectrometric characterization of flavonoids in extracts from *Passiflora incarnata. J Chromatogr A.* 1997;777(1):223–31.
19. Bokstaller S, Schmidt PC. A comparative study on the content of passionflower flavonoids and sesquiterpenes from valerian root extracts in pharmaceutical preparations by HPLC. *Pharmazie.* 1997;52(7):552–7.
20. Menghini A, Mancini LA. TLC determination of flavonoid accumulation in clonal populations of *Passiflora incarnata* L. *Pharmacol Res Commun.* 1988;20(Suppl. 5):113–6.

RED CLOVER

Description

Botanical name: *Trifolium pratense* L.

Common names: Cow clover, meadow clover, purple clover

Parts of plant used: Flowers, leaves, and stems

Uses: Treatment of age-related and hormone-dependent diseases including menopausal symptoms and osteoporosis.

Mode of Action

The isoflavone content in red clover was found to have estrogenic properties that may play an important role in moderation of menopausal symptoms and prevention of cancers as well as other health benefits.[1]

Chemical Markers

Various flavonoids and isoflavonoids as well as glycoside and glycoside malonate derivatives of flavonoids and isoflavonoids have been identified in red clover and related species. The major isoflavonoids include biochanin A, formononetin, sissotrin (biochanin A-7-O-glycoside), ononin (formononetin-7-O-glycoside), biochanin A-7-O-glycoside-6-O-malonate, formononetin-7-O-glycoside-6-malonate, and the minor isoflavonoids are daidzein, glycitein, calycosin, genistein, pratensein, pseudobaptigenin, irilone, prunetin, and their glycosides and glycoside malonates.

The identified flavonoids include quercetin, isoquercetin, hyperoside, apigenin, luteolin, apigenin-7-glycoside, and luteolin-7-glycoside.[1–4] Cyanogenic glycosides, caffeoyl derivatives, saponins, and sterols were also found in red clover.[5–7] The essential oils from flowers of red clover were studied by GC–MS and the main components were identified as maltol, linalool, 1-phenylethyl alcohol, phenol, phenylethyl acetate, acetophenone, and (Z)-3-hexenyl acetate.[8] As the isoflavonoids are believed to be the active components in red clover, they are used as marker compounds for quality control of red clover extracts.

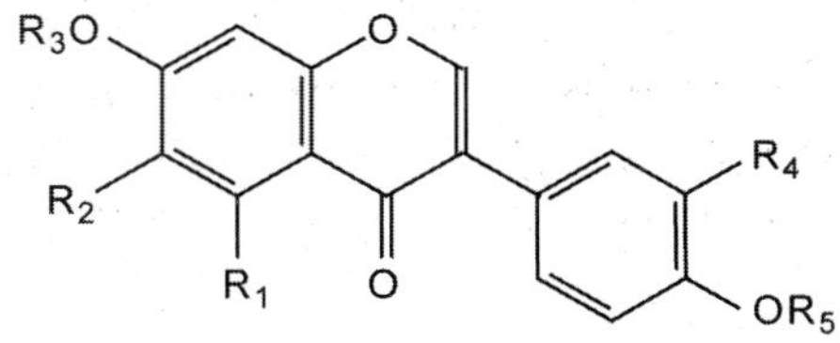

Name	R_1	R_2	R_3	R_4	R_5
Daidzein	H	H	H	H	H
Formononetin	H	H	H	H	Me
Genistein	OH	H	H	H	H
Pseudobaptigenin	H	H	H	1/M	OCH_2-
Biochanin A	OH	H	H	H	Me
Prunetin	OH	H	Me	H	H
Glycitein	H	OMe	H	H	H
Calycosin	H	H	H	OH	Me
Irilone	OH	1/M	OCH_2-	H	H
Pratensein	OH	H	H	OH	Me

Methods of Analysis

Several HPLC and LC–MS methods have been published to identify and analyze the isoflavones in red clover and red clover extracts. Due to the instabilities of isoflavone glycoside malonates, for quality control purposes, they should be converted to glycosides or converted to aglycones before analysis.

Method 1: The method of Lin et al.[4] was used. This method separates and identifies more than 30 compounds in red clover.

Sample preparation: For plant materials, extract about 0.5 g of flowers or 0.25 g of leaves with 10 mL of methanol–water (9:1) by sonication at room temperature for 60 minutes.

To get malonate-free samples, filter the resulting solution and heat in a sealed vial at 80°C to 85°C for 16 hours.

To get a hydrolyzed sample, filter, then mix 2 mL of the resulting solution with concentrated hydrochloric acid (37%, 0.4 mL), and heat in a sealed vial at 80°C to 85°C for 1.5 hours.

Chromatography

Column: Waters SymmetryShield, 5 µm, 150 × 3.9 mm with a guard column, (SymmetryShield, 5 µm, 3.9 × 20 mm).

Mobile phase: Solvent A = water containing 0.25% acetic acid, solvent B = acetonitrile containing 0.25% acetic acid.

Gradient: 14%B to 22%B in 36 minutes, then 22%B to 52%B in 64 minutes.

Flow rate: 0.2 mL/minute

Injection volume: 10 μL

Detection wavelength: 255 nm

Column temperature: 45°C

Validation data: Not available

Method 2: The method of Klejdus et al.[1] separates and identifies about 50 compounds in red clover.

Sample preparation: Extract about 0.5 g of material with methanol–water (7:3) using a magnetic stirrer and a "fex IKA Werke 50" extractor. Then clean up the sample using solid-phase extraction.

Chromatography

Column: Metachem Polaris C18A, 3 μm, 150 × 2.0 mm.

Mobile phase: Solvent A = water containing 0.2% acetic acid, solvent B = acetonitrile.

Gradient: 15%B to 25%B in 36 minutes, then 25%B to 55%B in 54 minutes, and finally 55%B to 15%B in 10 minutes.

Flow rate: 0.3 mL/minute

Injection volume: 10 μL

Detection wavelength: 255 nm

Column temperature: 40°C

Validation data: Not available

Method 3: The method of Krenn et al.[3] can be used to analyze the hydrolyzed aglycone daidzein, genistein, formononetin, and biochanin A in red clover.

Sample preparation: Extract 200 mg of pulverized drug with 30 mL of 80% methanol (acidified to pH 3 with trifluoroacetic acid) for 15 minutes under reflux at 85°C. Filter, and wash the residues with 20 mL of 80% methanol. Evaporate the extraction solution to dryness under reduced pressure, and dissolve the residue in 2 mL of dimethyl sulfoxide. To 500 μL of the dimethyl sulfoxide solution, add 40 μL of standard solution (15 mg of 6-methoxyflavanone/mL).

Chromatography

Column: Hypersil BDS C18, 5 μm, 250 × 4.0 mm.

Mobile phase: Solvent A = water (adjusted to pH 2.7 with sulfuric acid), solvent B = acetonitrile.

Gradient: 20%B to 37%B in 35 minutes, then 37%B to 100%B in 10 minutes, keep at 100%B for 10 minutes, then from 100%B to 20%B in 10 minutes, and keep at 20%B for 10 minutes.

Flow rate: 1 mL/minute

Injection volume: 10 µL

Detection wavelength: 254 nm

Validation data:

Linearity: 1.0 to 260, 1.5 to 260, 0.5 to 60, and 2.0 to 300 mg/L for daidzein, genistein, biochanin A, and formononetin, respectively, with correlation coefficients over 0.9988.

Accuracy: The percent recoveries were 99.2 for biochanin A and 98.2 for formononetin.

Precision: The RSD was less than 5.1% for all four compounds.

Selectivity: Peak identification was determined against standards.

Ruggedness: Not specified

Robustness: Not specified

LOD/LOQ: LOD = 1.6, 3.1, 0.6, and 3.7 ng for daidzein, genistein, biochanin A, and formononetin, respectively; LOQ = 5.0, 8.5, 2.0, and 10.0 for daidzein, genistein, biochanin A, and formononetin, respectively.

Method 4: The method of Wu et al.[2] identifies 31 isoflavones in red clover and also analyzes the hydrolyzed aglycone daidzein, genistein, formononetin, biochanin A, pseudobaptigenin, glycitein, calycosin, prunetin, irilone, and pratensein.

Sample preparation: For qualitative studies, extract about 100 mg of powder with 10 mL of 80% methanol using sonication for 1 hour.

For quantitative analysis of total aglycones, hydrolyze about 500 mg of herb powder with 50 mL of ethanol, 20 mL of water, and 8 mL of concentrated hydrochloric acid for 2 hours under nitrogen protection.

Chromatography

Column: Phenomenex Prodigy ODS3, 5 µm, 150 × 3.2 mm.

Mobile phase: Solvent A = water with 0.1% formic acid (vol/vol), solvent B = acetonitrile with 0.1% formic acid (vol/vol).

Gradient: 20%B to 40%B in 40 minutes.

Flow rate: 1 mL/minute

Injection volume: 5 µL

Detection wavelength: 254 nm

Validation data:

Linearity: 28.32 to 14,500, 32.23 to 16,500, 30.76 to 15,750, 21.97 to 11,250, 23.44 to 12,000, 25.39 to 1300, 25.39 to 1300, 25.39 to 1300, 23.44 to 12,000, and 23.44 to 12,000 ng/mL for daidzein, formononetin, genistein, pseudobaptigenin, glycitein, calycosin, prunetin, biochanin A, irilone, and pratensein, respectively, with correlation coefficients over 0.9995.

Accuracy: Not available

Precision: The RSD was less than 8% for all 10 aglycones at various concentrations.

Selectivity: Peak identification was determined against standards.

Ruggedness: Not specified

Robustness: Not specified

LOD/LOQ: LOQ = About 24 ng/mL for all 10 compounds

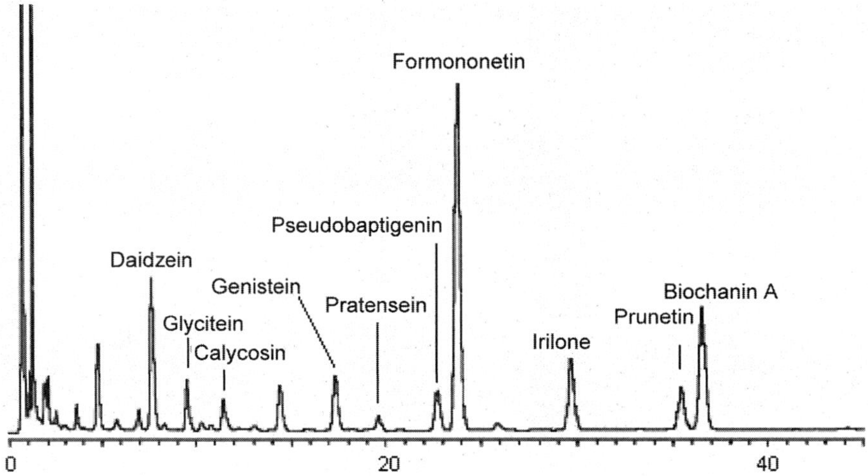

Representative HPLC chromatogram of red clover run by method 4.

References

1. Klejdus B, Vitamvasova-Sterbova D, Kuban V. Identification of isoflavone conjugates in red clover (*Trifolium pratense*) by liquid chromatography–mass spectrometry after two-dimensional solid-phase extraction. *Anal Chim Acta.* 2001;450(1–2):81–97.
2. Wu Q, Wang M, Simon JE. Determination of isoflavones in red clover and related species by high-performance liquid chromatography combined with ultraviolet and mass spectrometric detection. *J Chromatogr A.* 2003;1016(2):195–209.
3. Krenn L, Unterrieder I, Ruprechter R. Quantification of isoflavones in red clover by high-performance liquid chromatography. *J Chromatogr A.* 2002;777(1–2):123–8.
4. Lin LZ, He XG, Lindenmaier M, et al. LC–ESI-MS study of the flavonoid glycoside malonates of red clover (*Trifolium pratense*). *J Agric Food Chem.* 2000;48(2):354–65.

5. Oleszek W, Stochmal A. Triterpene saponins and flavonoids in the seeds of *Trifolium* species. *Phytochemistry.* 2002;61(2):165–70.
6. Popravko SA, Fraishtat PD, Sokolova SA, et al. Phytosterols and their glycosides in the roots of red clover (*Trifolium pratense* L.). *Prikladnaya Biokhimiya i Mikrobiologiya.* 1983;19(6):820–6.
7. Yoshihara T, Yoshikawa H, Kunimatsu S, et al. New amino acid derivatives conjugated with caffeic acid and DOPA from red clover (*Trifolium pratense*). *Agric Biol Chem.* 1977;41(9):1679–84.
8. Buchbauer G, Jirovetz L, Nikiforov A. Comparative investigation of essential clover flower oils from Austria using gas chromatography–flame ionization detection, gas chromatography–mass spectrometry, and gas chromatography–olfactometry. *J Agric Food Chem.* 1996;44(7):1827–8.

RHODIOLA

Description

Botanical name: *Rhodiola rosea*

Common names: Arctic root, golden root

Parts of plant used: Rhizomes

Uses: Improvement in mental health; as an adaptogenic, an antistress, and a cardioprotective agent.

Mode of Action

Rhodiola rosea extracts exhibited adaptogenic effects in mice and rabbits[1] and cardioprotective and antiadrenergic activities during stress.[2] An alcohol–water extract (1:1) was found to improve learning and long-term memory in mice.[3] One standardized extract, SHR-5, was reported to relieve stress-induced fatigue significantly in a double-blind cross-over study[4] and to improve capacity for mental work against a background of fatigue and stress.[5] But currently, no specific compound has been identified as responsible for these activities.

Chemical Markers

Phytochemistry study of *Rhodiola rosea* root has revealed the presence of several types of chemical compounds[6–8] including:

Phenylpropanoids [rosavin, rosin, rosarin, 4-methoxycinnamyl-O-β-glucopyranoside, cinnamyl-(6-β-xylopyranosyl)-O-β-D-glucopyranoside, cinnamyl-(6-α-arabinopyranosyl)-O-β-D-glucopyranoside].

Phenylethanol derivatives (salidroside, tyrosol), flavonoids (acetylrodalgin, kaempferol, kaempferol 7-rhamnoside, rodiolin, rodionin, rodiosin, tricin, tricin 5-glucoside, tricin 7-glucoside), monoterpenes (rosiridol, rosaridin), sterols (daucosterol, β-sitosterol), phenolic acids (chlorogenic acid, hydroxycinnamic acid, gallic acid), picein, and benzyl-O-β-D-glucopyranoside.

The essential oils of rhodiola rhizomes were found to contain decanol, geraniol, and 1,4-p-menthadien-7-ol as the most abundant volatiles.[9] Usually salidroside, rosavin, rosarin, rosin, and/or tyrosol are used as marker compounds for quality control of rhodiola, although they may not be the bioactive compounds.

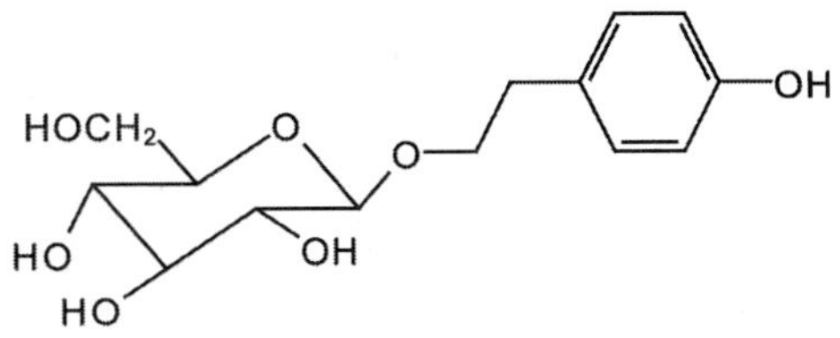

Salidroside

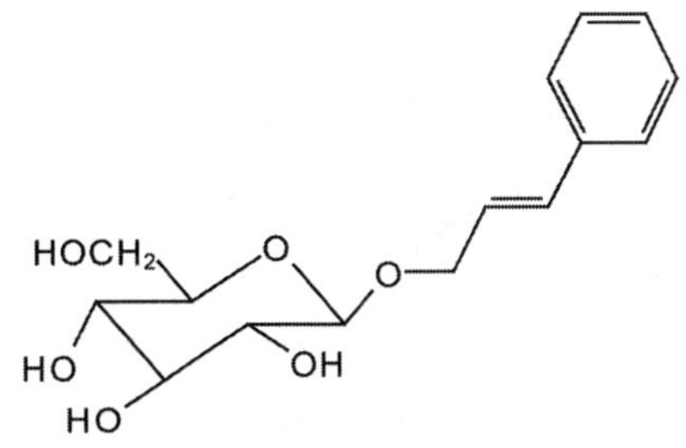

Rosin

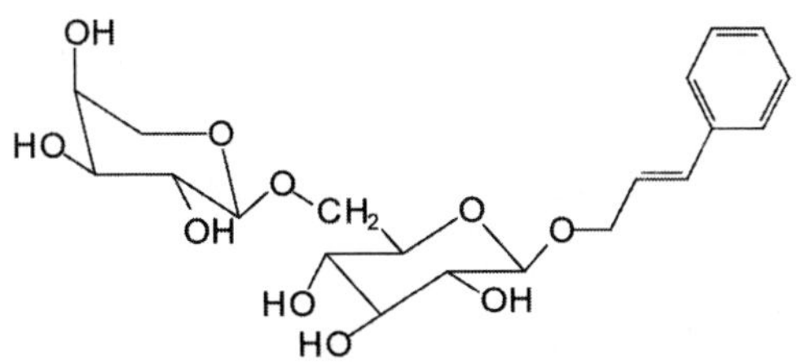

Rosavin

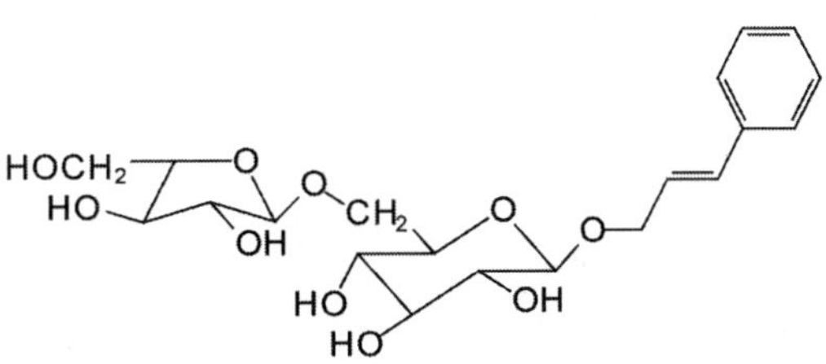

Rosarin

Marker compounds in *Rhodiola rosea*.

Methods of Analysis

Very few methods have been published for the analysis of chemicals in rhodiola, and most of the published methods only focused on the analysis of salidroside, not on rosavin, rosin, and rosarin because of the shortage of reference standards.

Method 1: The method of Ganzera et al.[10] can be used to analyze five compounds (salidroside, rosavin, rosarin, rosin, rosaridin) in rhodiola.

Sample preparation: Extract 1 g of the powdered root three times with 3 mL of methanol by sonication for 10 minutes. Centrifuge, combine the supernates, and dilute to a volume of 10 mL with methanol.

Chromatography

Column: Phenomenex Luna C18, 5 μm, 150 × 4.6 mm.

Mobile phase: Solvent A = 25 mM phosphate buffer adjusted to pH 7, solvent B = acetonitrile.

Gradient: 95%A/5%B to 80%A/20%B in 30 minutes.

Flow rate: 1.0 mL/minute

Injection volume: 10 μL

Detection wavelength: 205 nm

Column temperature: 60°C

Validation data:

Linearity: 16.5 to 500 mcg/mL with correlation coefficients over 0.9998 for all five compounds.

Accuracy: The percent recoveries were from 97.49 to 100.88 for these five compounds.

Precision: Not specified

Selectivity: Peak identification was determined against standards.

Ruggedness: Not specified

Robustness: Not specified

LOD/LOQ: LOD = 0.16 mcg/mL for rosavin and 0.62 mcg/mL for rosaridin.

Method 2: The method of Wang et al.[11] was used.

Sample preparation: Weigh 500 mg of root powder or 250 mg of root extract into a 50-mL volumetric flask, add 35 mL of 40% methanol aqueous solution, and sonicate for 45 minutes. Cool to room temperature and fill to volume with 40% methanol.

Chromatography

Column: Phenomenex Luna Phenylhexyl, 3 μm, 150 × 4.6 mm.

Mobile phase: Solvent A = 0.2% phosphoric acid, solvent B = acetonitrile.

Gradient: Initial 4%B, linear to 30%B in 20 minutes.

Flow rate: 1.2 mL/minute

Temperature: Ambient

Detection wavelength: 225 nm for 0 to 10 minutes and 254 nm for 10 to 20 minutes.

Injection volume: 10 μL

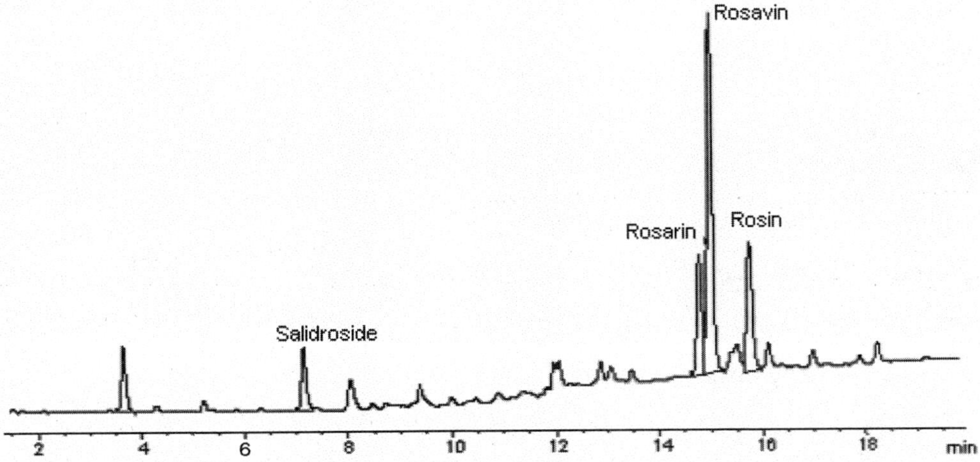

Representative HPLC chromatogram of *Rhodiola rosea* run by method 2.

References

1. Aksenova RA, Zotova MI, Nekhoda MF, et al. Stimulating and adaptogenic effects of a refined preparation of *Rhodiola rosea*; rhodosin. *Stimulyatory Tsent Nerv Sist*. 1966;77–9.
2. Maslova LV, Kondratyev BY, Maslov LN, et al. On the cardioprotective and antiadrenergic activity of *Rhodiola rosea* extract during stress. *Eksperimental'naya i Klinicheskaya Farmakologiya*. 1994;57(6):61–3.
3. Petkov VD, Yonkov D, Mosharoff A, et al. Effects of alcohol aqueous extract from *Rhodiola rosea* L. roots on learning and memory. *Acta Physiologica et Pharmacologica Bulgaria*. 1986;12(1):3–16.
4. Darbinyan V, Kteyan A, Panossian A, et al. *Rhodiola rosea* in stress-induced fatigue—a double-blind cross-over study of a standardized extract SHR-5 with a repeated low-dose regimen on the mental performance of healthy physicians during night duty. *Phytomedicine*. 2000;7(5):365–71.
5. Shevtsov VA, Zholus BI, Shervarly VI, et al. A randomized trial of two different doses of a SHR-5 *Rhodiola rosea* extract versus placebo and control of capacity for mental work. *Phytomedicine*. 2003;10(2–3):95–105.
6. Brown RP, Gerbarg PL, Ramazanov Z. *Rhodiola rosea:* A phytomedicinal overview. *HerbalGram*. 2002;56:40–52.
7. Zapesochnaya GG, Kurkin VA, Shchavlinskii AN. The chemical study of *Rhodiola rosea* L. *Int Conf Chem Biotechnol Biol Act Nat Prod*. [Proc.], 3rd 1987;4:404–8.
8. Wang LS, Wang L, Lu JJ, et al. Microwave technique extraction and content determination of polysaccharide in *Rhodiola rosea*. *Shihezi Daxue Xuebao, Ziran Kexueban*. 2002;6(1):18–9.
9. Rohloff J. Volatiles from rhizomes of *Rhodiola rosea* L. *Phytochemistry*. 2002;59(6):655–61.
10. Ganzera M, Yayla Y, Khan IA. Analysis of the marker compounds of *Rhodiola rosea* L. (golden root) by reversed-phase high-performance liquid chromatography. *Chem Pharm Bull*. 2001;49(4):465–7.
11. Wang M, Jin Y, Wu QL, et al. Chemistry, pharmacology and quality control of selected popular oriental herbs in the U.S. market. *Asian Functional Foods*. 2004, in press.

SCHISANDRA

Description

Botanical name: *Schisandra chinensis*

Common name: Wu-Wei-Zi

Parts of plant used: Berries

Uses: Liver protection, as an adaptogen.

Mode of Action

A berry extract standardized with total lignans was pharmacologically and clinically proven to be a good liver protective herb. In China, a clinical trial with more than 5000 patients having different types of hepatitis was performed in the 1980s. The patients were treated with a schisandra fruits preparation. The elevated GPT (glutamic pyruvic transaminase, an enzyme found primarily in the liver, which is released into the bloodstream as the result of liver damage) level returned to normal with 75% of patients after they were treated for 20 days with schisandra.[1] Schisandra was also found to improve physical performance and was used to prevent and to treat neurodegenerative diseases.[2]

Chemical Markers

Schisandra chinensis is a rich source of lignans. More than 30 lignans have been purified from it with schisandrol A (other names: schisandrin, wuweizi alcohol A, wuweizichun A), schisandrin B (γ-schisandrin, wuweizisu B), schisandrol B (gomisin A, wuweizi alcohol B, wuweizichun B), schisandrin A (deoxyschisandrin, wuweizisu A), schisantherin A (gomisin C, wuweizi ester A), and schisantherin B (gomisin B, wuweizi ester B) as the major ones.[3]

Several other type of chemicals including daucosterol, 5-hydroxymethyl-2-furancarboxaldehyde, 2-methyl citrate, protocatechuic acid, quinic acid, thymoquinol 2-glucoside, thymoquinol 5-glucoside, and zingerone glucoside were also identified in the fruits of *Schisandra chinensis*.[4]

The essential oil of schisandra was found to be composed mainly of terpenes with copaene, alpha-farnesene, and alpha-cubebene as the major constituents.[5] As the lignans have been proven clinically to be the bioactive components in schisandra, they are used as chemical markers for quality control.

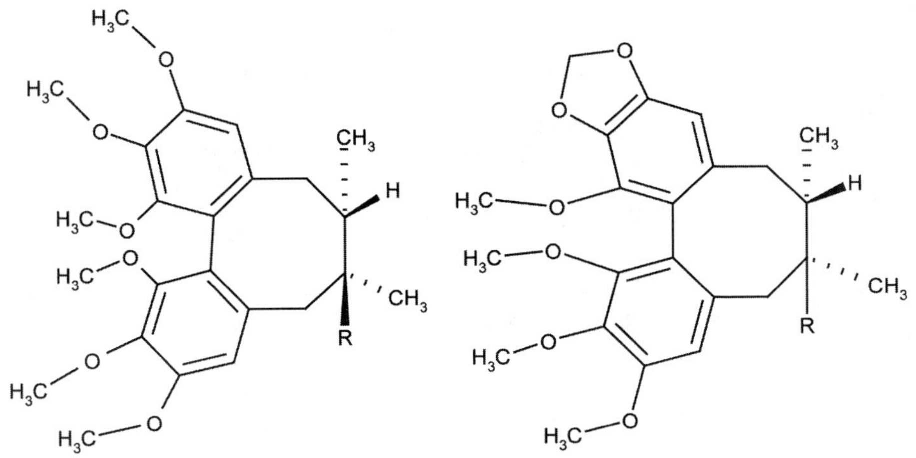

Schisandrol A: R = OH
Schisandrin A: R = H

Schisandrol B: R = OH
Schisandrin B: R = H

Four major lignans in schisandra.

Methods of Analysis

Various methods have been used to analyze the lignan content in schisandra, with HPLC being the most acceptable approach. Most of the published HPLC methods use a methanol–water or acetonitrile–water isocratic mobile phase and offer good separation, while a gradient mobile phase provides a little better separation. The detection wavelength was usually 254 nm. As schisandra lignans are fat-soluble compounds, GC is a good alternative.[6] Capillary electrochromatography and micellar electrokinetic capillary chromatography also have been used to analyze lignans in schisandra.[7]

Extraction is of key importance for accurate analysis of lignans in schisandra. Generally, pure methanol is a good solvent for extracting samples for analysis.

Method 1: The method of Bartlova et al.[8] can be used to analyze the six major lignans: schisandrol A, schisandrol B, schisandrin A, schisandrin B, gomisin N, and schisandrin C. Their method used two chromatographic sets and columns.

Sample preparation: Initally, use supercritical fluid extraction, then dissolve the samples in methanol for analysis. Or extract 0.5 g of sample with 95% ethanol by refluxing for 0.5 hour, then dissolve in acetonitrile–water (85:15).

Chromatography

Column 1: Nucleosil 100, 5 μm, C18 endcapped EC 250 × 4.0 mm.

Mobile phase: Solvent A = water, solvent B = acetonitrile.

Gradient:

Time (minutes)	%A	%B
0	50	50
5	50	50
35	40	60
55	30	70
70	30	70

Or mobile phase: Solvent A = water, solvent B = methanol.
Gradient:

Time (minutes)	%A	%B
0	30	70
1	30	70
35	5	95
40	5	95

Flow rate: 0.75 mL/minute
Injection volume: 20 μL
Detection wavelength: 254 nm
Column temperature: Ambient
Column 2: Merck-LiChrospher 100 RP-18, 5 μm, 250 × 4.0 mm.
Mobile phase: Solvent A = water, solvent B = acetonitrile.
Gradient:

Time (minutes)	%A	%B
0	60	40
60	30	70
90	30	70

Flow rate: 0.5 mL/minute
Injection volume: 20 μL
Detection wavelength: 254 nm
Column temperature: 25°C

Validation data: Not available

Method 2: The method of Wang et al.[3] was used.

Sample preparation: Weigh the dried schisandra fruits and fruit extracts (9:1) (400 mg for fruit powders and 200 mg for extract) into a 100-mL volumetric flask. Add 70 mL of methanol and sonicate for 30 minutes, then cool to room temperature, and fill to volume with methanol.

Chromatography

Column: Phenomenex Luna C18(2), 5 μm, 250 × 4.6 mm.

Mobile phase: Solvent A = water (0.1% formic acid), solvent B = acetonitrile.

Gradient:

Time (minutes)	%A	%B
0	55	45
12	40	60
24	40	60
40	10	90
45	10	90

Flow rate: 1.0 mL/minute

Injection volume: 10 μL

Detection wavelength: 255 nm

Column temperature: Ambient

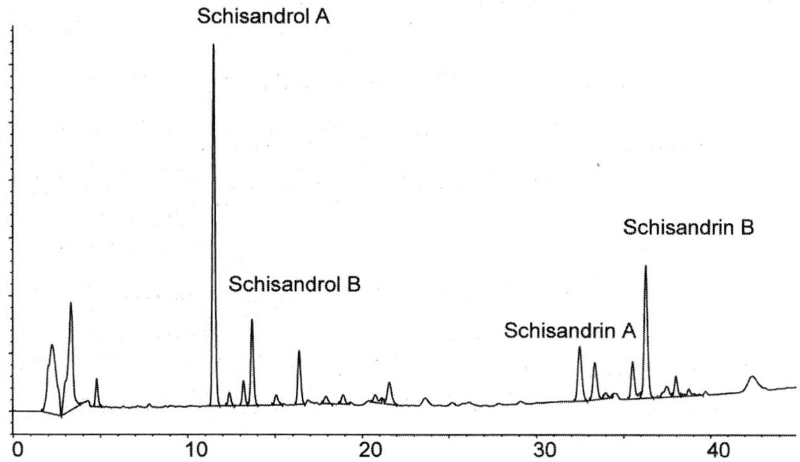

Representative HPLC chromatogram of schisandra run by method 2.

References

1. Chang HM, But PH. Pharmacology and application of Chinese materia medica. Singapore: *World Science*; 1986:1:773.
2. Hanche JL, Burgos RA, Ahumada F. *Schisandra chinensis* (Turcz.) Baillon *Fitoterapia.* 1999;70:451–71.
3. Wang M, Wu QL, Tadmor Y, et al. *Schisandra chinensis*: Chemistry and analysis. In: *ACS symposium series 859: oriental foods and herbs, chemistry and health effects.* Washington, DC: American Chemical Society; 2003:234–46.
4. Dai H, Zhou J, Peng Z, et al. Studies on chemical constituents of *Schisandra chinensis. Tianran Chanwu Yanjiu Yu Kaifa.* 2001;13(1):24–6.
5. Qin B, Tian Z, Lou Z. Constituents of the volatile oil from the fruit of *Schisandra chinensis. Yaoxue Tongbao.* 1988;23(6):338–9.

6. Sohn HJ, Bock JY, Baik SO, et al. Determination of lignan compounds in fruits of *Schisandra chinensis* Baillon by capillary-GC(FID). *Han'guk Nonghwa Hakhoechi.* 1989;32(4):350–6.
7. Sterbova H, Sevcikova P, Kvasnickova L, et al. Determination of lignans in *Schisandra chinensis* using micellar electrokinetic capillary chromatography. *Electrophoresis.* 2002;23(2):253–8.
8. Bartlova M, Opletal L, Chobot V, et al. Liquid chromatographic analysis of supercritical carbon dioxide extracts of *Schizandra chinensis*. *J Chromatogr B.* 2002;770(1–2):283–9.

SENNA

Description

Botanical names: *Cassia angustifolia* Vahl, *Cassia acutifolia* Delile, *Senna alexandrina* Mill., *Cassia senna* L.

Common names: Alexandrian senna, Indian senna, Tinnevelly senna

Parts of plant used: Leaves and pods

Uses: As a laxative.

Mode of Action

Senna is widely used as a herbal laxative. Sennosides, diglucosides of sennidins, are the purgative principles of this plant. Sennosides are metabolized to anthrones and anthranoles in the human intestine. The interaction between anthrones and immune cells of the colon has been suggested to be the basis for its laxative activity.[1,2]

Chemical Markers

The active components in senna leaves were first identified as sennosides A and B (dimeric products of emodin and/or rhein), which, when hydrolyzed, give the aglycones sennidins A and B and two molecules of glucose. Later work demonstrated the presence of sennosides C and D, small quantities of monomeric glycosides, and free anthraquinones. The active constituents of the pods are similar to those of the leaves but in larger quantities. Other compounds such as flavonoids and sterols have also been isolated from senna. The major flavonoids were found to be diglucosides of quercetin, kaempferol, and isorhamnetin.[3,4] Recently, three unique compounds, tinnevellin-8-glucoside, cassiaphenone A-2-glucoside, and cassiaphenone B-2-glucoside, were identified in senna.[3] Sennosides A and B are used as the marker compounds for quality control of senna products.

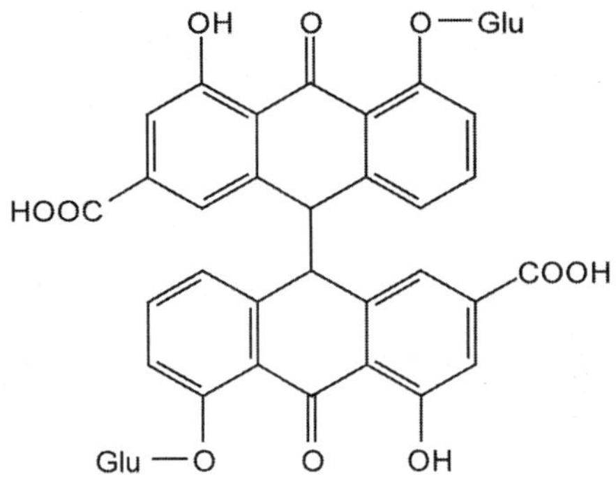

Sennoside A

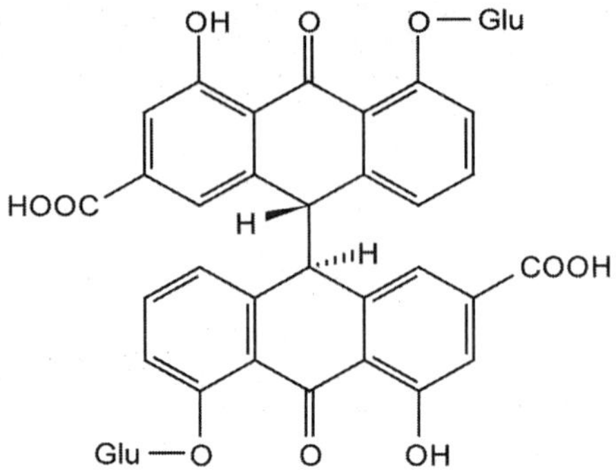

Sennoside B

Methods of Analysis

Various methods have been used to analyze sennosides A and B for quality control of senna, including fluorometry, spectrophotometry, HPLC, and capillary electrophoresis.[2,5–7] Currently, the United States Pharmacopeia uses a fluorometric method to analyze the active components in senna preparations, but this method can determine only the total amount of dianthrone and anthraquinone glucosides and does not provide a detailed analysis.

Method 1: The method of Bala et al.[5] was used.

Sample preparation: Powder 1 g of leaves and extract with hexane (3 × 25 mL); discard the hexane extracts. Extract the remains with 25 mL of methanol–water (7:3) overnight at room temperature, then extract with methanol–water (7:3) (2 × 25 mL). Combine the extraction solutions and dilute to 100 mL with methanol– water (7:3).

Chromatography

Column: Waters Symmetry C18, 5 µm, 150 × 4.6 mm.

Mobile phase: Solvent A = methanol–water–acetic acid (20:80:0.1 vol/vol/vol, pH 4), solvent B = methanol–water–acetic acid (80:20:0.1 vol/vol/vol, pH 4).

Gradient:

Time (minutes)	%A	%B
0	80	20
5	80	20
25	0	100
35	0	100
40	80	20

Flow rate: 0.6 mL/minute for the first 20 minutes, increasing to 1.0 mL/minute at 30 minutes.

Injection volume: 10 µL

Detection wavelength: 285 nm

Column temperature: 25°C

Validation data:

Linearity: 2 to 50 mcg for sennosides A and B.

Accuracy: Not specified

Precision: Not specified

Selectivity: Peak identification was determined against standards.

Ruggedness: Not specified

Robustness: Not specified

LOD/LOQ: 0.2 mcg/mL for sennoside A and 0.1 mcg/mL for sennoside B.

Method 2: The method of Sun and Su[8] was used.

Sample preparation: Grind 10 tablets of senna preparation to powder. Dissolve 5 to 15 mg in 5 mL of sodium bicarbonate solution (1 g in 1000 mL of water).

Chromatography

Column: Phenomenex Hypersil C18, 5 μm, 250 × 4.6 mm.

Mobile phase: pH 6 acetate buffer (prepared using 1 M sodium acetate and 1 M acetic acid). This buffer was diluted 10 times and mixed together with acetonitrile (70:30 vol/vol). To 1000 mL of the mixed solution, 2.17 g of tetrahexylammonium bromide was added, and the resulting solution was used as the mobile phase.

Flow rate: 1.0 mL/minute

Injection volume: 20 μL

Detection wavelength: 275 nm

Column temperature: 40°C

Validation data:

Linearity: 30 to 70 mcg/mL for sennosides A and B with correlation coefficients over 0.9997.

Accuracy: The percent recoveries were 101.73 and 101.81 for sennosides A and B, respectively.

Precision: The RSD was less than 0.4%.

Selectivity: Peak identification was determined against standards.

Ruggedness: Not specified

Robustness: Not specified

LOD/LOQ: Not specified

Method 3: The unpublished method of Mingfu Wang was used.

Sample preparation: Add 100 mg of herb powder or extract to a 50-mL volumetric flask, and add 35 mL of water. Sonicate for 40 minutes, and shake for 20 minutes. Cool the sample to room temperature, and fill to volume.

Chromatography

Column: Phenomenex Luna Phenylhexyl, 3 μm, 150 × 4.6 mm.

Mobile phase: Solvent A = water (0.2% phosphoric acid), solvent B = acetonitrile.

Gradient: 10%B to 30%B in 20 minutes, then wash with 90%B for 10 minutes.

Flow rate: 1.0 mL/minute

Injection volume: 10 μL

Detection wavelength: 360 nm

Column temperature: Ambient

Validation data: Not available

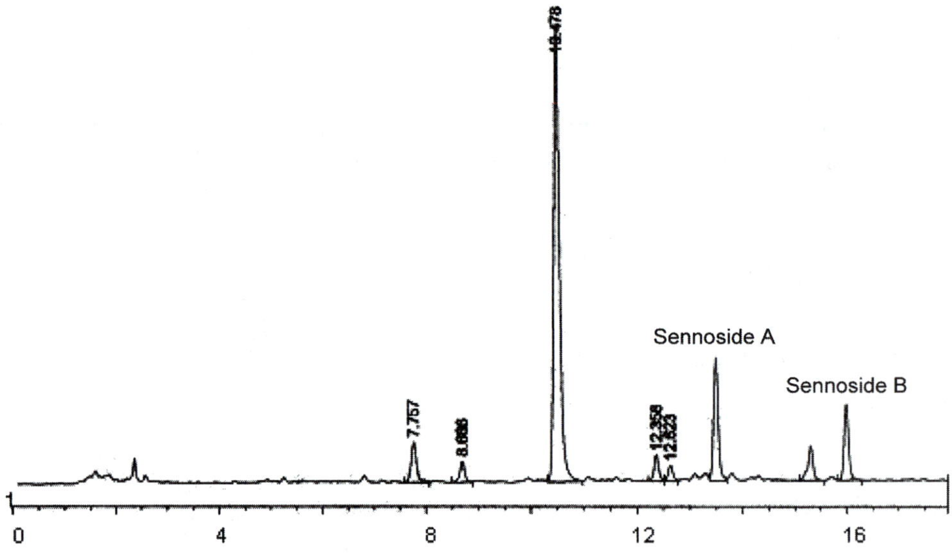

Representative HPLC chromatogram of senna run by method 3.

References

1. Lemli J. The mode of action of the sennosides. *Bull Acad Natl Med*. 1995;179(8):1605–11.
2. Djozan DJ, Assadi Y. Determination of anthraquinones in rhubarb roots, dock flowers, and senna leaves by normal-phase high-performance liquid chromatography. *Talanta*. 1995;42(6):861–5.
3. Terreaux C, Wang Q, Ioset JR, et al. Complete LC/MS analysis of a *Tinnevelli senna* pod extract and subsequent isolation and identification of two new benzophenone glucosides. *Planta Med*. 2002;68(4):349–54.

4. Franz G. The senna drug and its chemistry. *Pharmacology.* 1993;47(S1):2–6.
5. Bala S, Uniyal GC, Dubey T, et al. An improved method for the analysis of sennosides in *Cassia angustifolia* by high-performance liquid chromatography. *Phytochem Anal.* 2001;12(4):277–80.
6. Weng WC, Sheu SJ. Separation of anthraquinones by capillary electrophoresis and high-performance liquid chromatography. *J High Resolut Chromatogr.* 2000;23(2):143–8.
7. Sugiyama A, Nakashima M, Nishida S. Rapid analysis of sennosides A and B in health teas by capillary electrophoresis. *J Health Sci.* 1999;45(5):293–6.
8. Sun SW, Su HT. Validated HPLC method for determination of sennosides A and B in senna tablets. *J Pharm Biomed Anal.* 2002;29(5):881–94.

SIBERIAN GINSENG (ELEUTHERO)

Description

Botanical names: *Eleutherococcus senticosus* Maxim; *Acanthopanax senticosus* Harms

Common names: Ci-Wu-Jia, Eleuthero, Ussurian thorny pepperbush

NOTE: *Eleutherococcus senticosus* (Eleuthero) is often referred to as "Siberian Ginseng." It is not related to Asian or American ginseng, however.

Parts of plant used: Roots

Uses: As an adaptogen; immune-enhancing agent; a remedy for stress, fatigue, and depression.

Mode of Action

Several clinical trials have been performed to validate the activity of Siberian ginseng. The results are not consistent: some results showed that Siberian ginseng or a herbal formula with Siberian ginseng was effective, and some results were negative.[1–4] Currently, no active components have been identified in Siberian ginseng.

Chemical Markers

Several types of compounds have been identified in Siberian ginseng roots and leaves including polysaccharides, phenolics (coumarins, phenylpropanoic derivatives, lignans), sterols and triterpene glycosides, thymidine, and isomaltol 3-O-α-D-glucopyranoside.[5–12] Most of the compounds isolated from Siberian ginsengs were named as eleutherosides, although they are different types of compounds. For example, eleutheroside A (daucosterol) is a sterol, eleutheroside B (syringin) is a phenylpropanoic derivative, eleutheroside B1 (isofraxetin) is a coumarin glycoside, eleutheroside E is a lignan diglycoside, eleutheroside E1 is a lignan monoglycoside, and eleutheroside I is a triterpene saponin. Because no bioactive components have been identified in Siberian ginseng, and eleutherosides B and E are the major phenolic compounds in the root extract, they are used as marker compounds for quality control of Siberian ginseng extract. Usually in the market, Siberian ginseng is sold as a 0.8% extract of eleutherosides B and E.

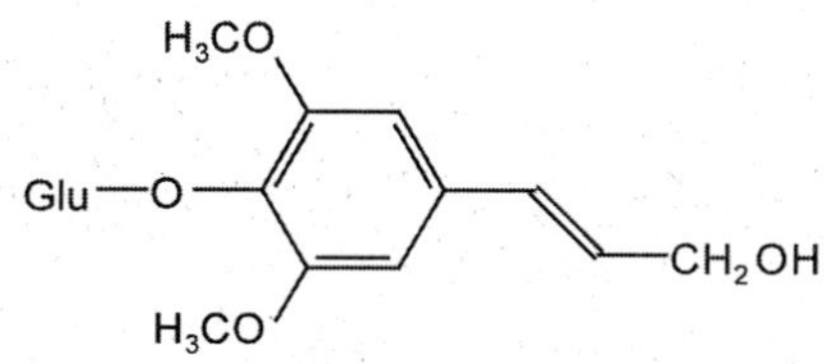

Eleutheroside B

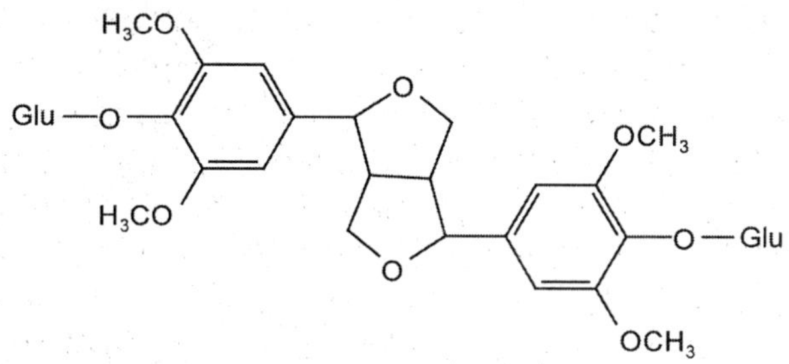

Eleutheroside E

Major phenolics in Siberian ginseng.

Methods of Analysis

The compounds in Siberian ginseng root have been analyzed by various methods including TLC, HPLC, LC–MS, and micellar electrokinetic chromatography.[13–16] HPLC is the most popular method and has been widely used in the industry for analysis of eleutherosides B and E as a way of quality control of Siberian ginseng extract.

Extraction is key for accurate analysis of phytochemicals. Usually, methanol–water solutions are suitable extraction solvents.

Method 1: The method found at www.nsfina.org was used.

Sample preparation: For root powder, transfer about 2 g to a 100-mL round-bottom flask, and reflux with 50 mL of methanol–water (60:40) for 30 minutes. Filter the extraction solution into a 100-mL volumetric flask. Extract the residue a second time for 30 minutes using 50 mL of the same solvent, and add to the first extraction solution. Dilute to volume with methanol–water (60:40).

For powdered extracts, weigh about 75 mg into a 25-mL volumetric flask. Add 20 mL of methanol–water (60:40), and sonicate, with occasional shaking, for 30 minutes. Cool, and dilute to volume with methanol–water (60:40).

Chromatography

Column: Phenomenex Luna C18, 5 μm, 250 × 4.6 mm or YMC-Pack Pro C18, 250 × 4.6 mm (an equivalent column).

Mobile phase: Solvent A = water (adjusted to pH 2 with phosphoric acid), solvent B = acetonitrile.

Gradient:

Time (minutes)	%A	%B
0	90	10
2	90	10
20	70	30
25	70	30
27	90	10
45	90	10

Column temperature: 40°C

Flow rate: 0.8 mL/minute

Detection wavelength: 215 nm

Injection volume: 20 μL

Validation data: Not available, but this method is known to be a fully validated method.

Method 2: The method at www.chromadex.com was used.

Sample preparation: Add about 1 g of Siberian ginseng extract to a 100-mL volumetric flask. Add 50 mL of 10% acetonitrile, and shake until the extract is dissolved. Dilute to volume with 10% acetonitrile.

Chromatography

Column: Phenomenex Luna C18(2), 3 μm, 150 × 4.6 mm.

Mobile phase: Solvent A = water–acetonitrile (90:10), solvent B = water–acetonitrile (60:40).

Gradient: 100%A to 100%B in 25 minutes

Flow rate: 1.0 mL/minutes.

Injection volume: 20 μL

Detection wavelength: 220 nm

Method 3: The method of Yat et al.[17] was used.

Sample preparation: Extract powdered root samples at 60°C with 20% aqueous methanol (2 × 30 mL) for 30 minutes each. Evaporate the combined extracts to dryness, and dissolve in aqueous 0.05% trifluoroacetic acid–methanol (1:4).

Chromatography

Column: Beckman Ultrasphere ODS, 5 μm, 250 × 4.6 mm, with a Beckman ODS precolumn, 5 μm, 45 × 4.6 mm.

Mobile phase: Solvent A = water (0.05% trifluoroacetic acid), solvent B = acetonitrile.

Gradient: 10%B to 50%B in 30 minutes.

Flow rate: 1.0 mL/minute

Injection volume: 20 μL

Detection wavelength: 220 nm

Column temperature: Ambient

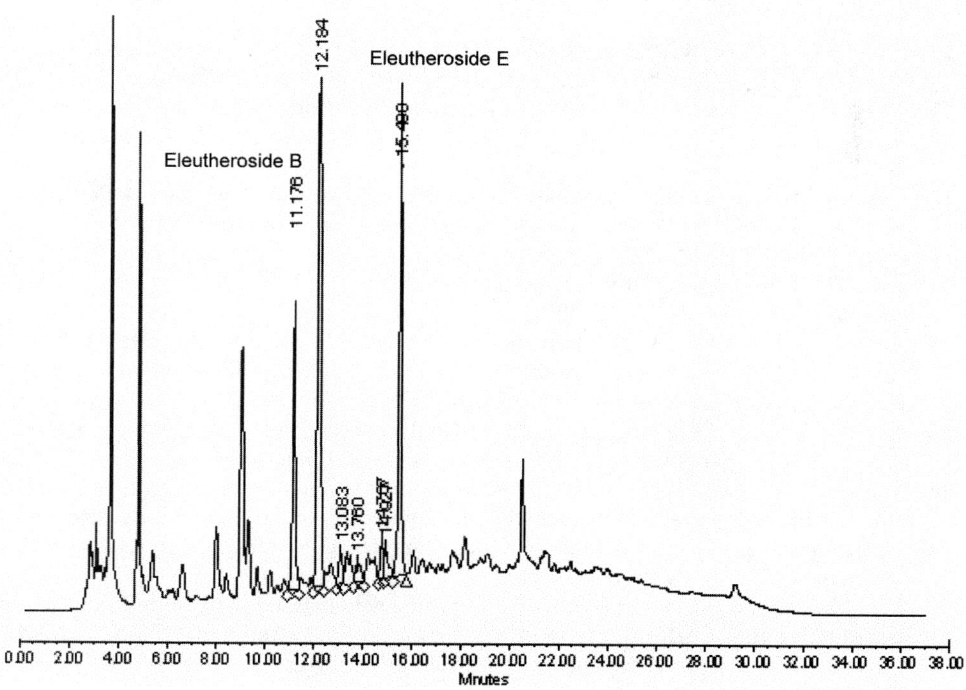

Representative HPLC chromatogram of Siberian ginseng extract run by method 1 using Phenomenex Luna C18(2) column.

References

1. Amaryan G, Astvatsatryan V, Gabrielyan E, et al. Double-blind, placebo-controlled, randomized, pilot clinical trial of ImmunoGuard—a standardized fixed combination of *Andrographis paniculata* Nees, with *Eleutherococcus senticosus* Maxim, *Schizandra chinensis* Bail and *Glycyrrhiza glabra* L. extracts in patients with Familial Mediterranean Fever. *Phytomedicine.* 2003;10(4):271–85.
2. Panossian A, Davtyan T, Gukassyan N, et al. Effect of andrographolide and Kan Jang—fixed combination of extract SHA-10 and extract SHE-3—on proliferation of human lymphocytes, production of cytokines and immune activation markers in the whole blood cells culture. *Phytomedicine.* 2002;9(7):598–605.
3. Gaffney BT, Hugel HM, Rich PA. The effects of *Eleutherococcus senticosus* and *Panax ginseng* on steroidal hormone indices of stress and lymphocyte subset numbers in endurance athletes. *Life Sci.* 2001;70(4):431–42.
4. Szolomicki S, Samochowiec L, Wojcicki J, et al. The influence of active components of *Eleutherococcus senticosus* on cellular defence and physical fitness in man. *Phytother Res.* 2000;14(1):30–5.
5. Li XC, Barnes DL, Khan IA. A new lignan glycoside from *Eleutherococcus senticosus. Planta Med.* 2001;67(8):776–8.
6. Tolonen A, Joutsamo T, Mattlla S, et al. Identification of isomeric dicaffeoylquinic acids from *Eleutherococcus senticosus* using HPLC-ESI/TOF/MS and 1H-NMR methods. *Phytochem Anal.* 2002;13(6):316–28.
7. Makarieva TN, Dmitrenok AS, Stonik VA, et al. Lignans from *Eleutherococcus senticosus* (Siberian ginseng). *Pharm Sci.* 1997;3(10):525–7.
8. Kurkin VA, Zapesochnaya GG, Vandyshev VV. Phenolic compounds from *Eleutherococcus senticosus. Khimiya Prirodnykh Soedinenii.* 1991;(6):854–6.
9. Hikino H, Takahashi M, Otake K, et al. Isolation and hypoglycemic activity of eleutherans A, B, C, D, E, F, and G: glycans of *Eleutherococcus senticosus* roots. *J Nat Prod.* 1986; 49(2):293–7.
10. Frolova GM, Ovodov YS. Triterpenoid glycosides of *Eleutherococcus senticosus* leaves. II. Structure of eleutherosides I, K, L, and M. *Khimiya Prirodnykh Soedinenii.* 1971;(5):618–22.
11. Ovodov YS, Frolova GM, Nefedova MY, et al. Glycosides of *Eleutherococcus senticosus.* II. The structure of eleutherosides A, B1, C, and D. *Khimiya Prirodnykh Soedinenii.* 1967; 3(1):63–4.
12. Ovodov YS, Frolova GM, Dzizenko AK, et al. Structure and properties of eleutheroside B, glycoside of *Eleutherococcus senticosus.* Izvestiya Akademii Nauk SSSR, *Seriya Khimicheskaya.* 1969(6):1370–2.
13. Choi YH, Kim J. Quantitative analysis of eleutherosides B and E using HPLC–ESI/MS. *Saengyak Hakhoechi.* 2002;33(2):88–91.
14. Zgorka G, Kawka S. Application of conventional UV, photodiode array (PDA) and fluorescence (FL) detection to analysis of phenolic acids in plant material and pharmaceutical preparations. *J Pharm Biomed Anal.* 2001;24(5–6):1065–72.
15. Pietta PG, Mauri PL, Gardana C, et al. Micellar electrokinetic chromatographic/ultraviolet diode array analysis of *Eleutherococcus senticosus. Phytochem Anal.* 1994;5(6):305–8.
16. Vanhaelen M, Vanhaelen-Fastre R. Quantitative determination of biologically active constituents in crude extracts of medicinal plants by thin-layer chromatography-densitometry. II. *Eleutherococcus senticosus* Maxim., *Panax ginseng* Meyer and *Picrorrhiza kurroa* Royle. *J Chromatogr A.* 1984;312:497–503.
17. Yat PN, Arnason JT, Awang Dennis VC. An improved extraction procedure for the rapid, quantitative high-performance liquid chromatographic estimation of the main eleutherosides (B and E) in *Eleutherococcus senticosus* (Eleuthero). *Phytochem Anal.* 1998;9(6): 291–5.

SKULLCAP

Description

Botanical name: *Scutellaria baicalensis* Georgi

Common names: Chinese skullcap, Huang-Qin

Parts of plant used: Dried roots

Uses: Treatment of upper respiratory infections, as an anti-inflammatory agent.

Mode of Action

Few clinical trials have involved the herb skullcap alone. However, clinical trials have tested herbal formulas that included skullcap as one of the main ingredients. The total flavonoids, especially baicalin, baicalein, wogonin, and wogonin 7-O-glucuronide, are believed to be the active ingredients in skullcap, and various in vitro and in vivo experiments have established the activity of these compounds.[1–3]

Chemical Markers

Skullcap contains high amounts of flavonoids in the roots. Four flavones (baicalin, baicalein, wogonin, wogonin 7-O-glucuronide) are the major components. Other identified flavones include apigenin, apigenin 7-O-glucuronide, baicalin methyl ester, chrysin 6-C-β-D-glucopyranoside, chrysin 8-C-β-D-glucopyranoside, chrysin 7-O-β-D-glucuronopyranoside, chrysin 6-C-β-D-glucoside-8-C-α-L-arabinoside, isoscutellarein, isoscutellarein 8-O-glucuronide, 6,2′-dihydroxy-5,7,8,6′-tetramethoxyflavone, oroxylin A, oroxylin A glucuronide, 3,5,7,2′,6′-pentahydroxyflavanone, salvigenin, scutellarein, skullcapflavone II, 5,7,2′,6′-tetrahydroxyflavone, 5,7,2′,5′-tetrahydroxyflavone, 5,7,2′,5′-tetrahydroxy-8,6′-dimethoxyflavone, 5,2′,6′-trihydroxy-6,7-dimethoxyflavone 2′-O-glucoside, 5,7,2′-trihydroxy-6-methoxyflavone 7-O-β-D-glucuronopyranoside, and 5,2′,6′-trihydroxy-6,7,8-trimethoxyflavone 2′-O-glucoside.[4–6]

Flavanones (hydrobaicalin, carthamidin 7-O-glucuronide, isocarthamidin 7-O-glucuronide), lignans [(+)-5,5′-dimethoxylariciresinol, hedyotol C-4-O-β-glucopyranoside, hedyotol D-4-O-β-glucopyranoside, *erythro*-guaiacylglycerol-β-syringaresinol ether 4-O-β-glucopyranoside], phenylethanoids, phenylpropanoids, and sterols also were isolated from skullcap.[5–9] Usually, the four major flavonoids (baicalin, baicalein, wogonin, wogonin 7-O-glucuronide) are used as marker compounds for quality control of skullcap.

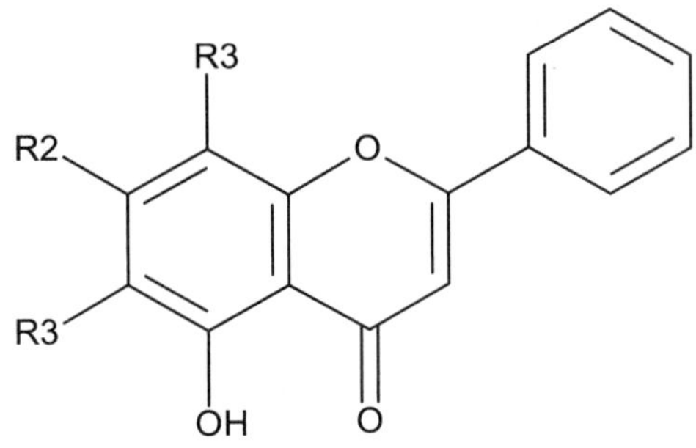

Baicalein: R_1 = H, R_2 = OH, R_3 = OH
Baicalin: R_1 = H, R_2 = O-glucuronyl, R_3 = OH
Wogonin: R_1 = OCH_3, R_2 = OH, R_3 = H
Wogonin-7-glucuronide: R_1 = OCH_3, R_2 = O-glucuronyl, R_3 = H
Oroxylin A: R_1 = H, R_2 = OH, R_3 = OCH_3
Oroxylin A-7-glucuronide: R_1 = H, R_2 = O-glucuronyl, R_3 = OCH_3

Major flavonoids in skullcap.

Methods of Analysis

Various HPLC methods have been published for analysis of the flavonoids in skullcap and related species.[10–13] Colorimetric methods and micellar electrokinetic chromatography also have been used to analyze the flavonoids in skullcap.[14] The flavonoids in skullcap can be extracted easily with aqueous alcohol–acetonitrile solution.

Method 1: The method of Takino et al.[15] provides clear separation for six flavonoids (baicalin, baicalein, wogonin, wogonin 7-O-glucuronide, oroxylin, and oroxylin 7-glucuronide).

Sample preparation: Extract about 2.5 g of root powder with 50 mL of 30% acetonitrile for 1 hour at 60°C to 70°C and repeat the procedure three times. Adjust the volume to 250 mL with 30% aqueous acetonitrile solution.

Chromatography

Column: Waters NovaPak C18 Radial-pak, 100 × 8.0 mm.

Mobile phase: Solvent A = methanol–acetic acid–water (5:5:90), solvent B = methanol–acetic acid–water (90:5:5).

Gradient: 40%B to 80%B in 40 minutes.

Flow rate: 1.0 mL/minute

Injection volume: 10 μL

Detection wavelength: 275 nm

Validation data: Not available

Method 2: The method of Bochorakova et al.[16] was used.

Sample preparation: Not available

Chromatography

Column: Separon SGX C18, 5 µm, 150 × 3.0 mm.

Mobile phase: Solvent A = water–acetonitrile (20:80), solvent B = water–acetonitrile (40:60). The water contained 0.1 mol of triethylamine and the pH was adjusted to 2.5 with phosphoric acid.

Gradient:

Time (minutes)	%A	%B
0	70	30
1	70	30
16	0	100
25	0	100

Flow rate: 0.5 mL/minute

Injection volume: 10 µL

Detection wavelength: 270 nm

Validation data:

Linearity: 5 to 50 mg/L for wogonin 7-O-glucuronide with a correlation coefficient of 0.9971 and 5 to 50 mg/L for baicalin with a correlation coefficient of 0.9987.

Accuracy: Not specified

Precision: Not specified

Selectivity: Peak identification was determined against standards.

Ruggedness: Not specified

Robustness: Not specified

LOD/LOQ: Not specified

Method 3: The unpublished method of Mingfu Wang was used.

Sample preparation: Transfer about 100 mg of skullcap powder to a 50-mL volumetric flask, add 35 mL of extraction solvent (60% methanol), and sonicate for 45 minutes. Cool to room temperature and fill to volume with 60% methanol.

Chromatography

Column: Phenomenex Luna Phenylhexyl, 3 µm, 150 × 4.6 mm with Phenomenex Phenylhexyl guard cartridge.

Mobile phase: Solvent A = water (0.1% formic acid by volume), solvent B = acetonitrile (0.1% formic acid by volume), solvent C = isopropanol.

Gradient:

Time (minutes)	%A	%B	%C
0	84	14	2
6	84	14	2
10	78	20	2
20	78	20	2
40	58	40	2
50	38	60	2

Flow rate: 1.0 mL/minute

Injection volume: 5 μL

Detection wavelength: 275 nm

Column temperature: 40°C

Validation data: Not available

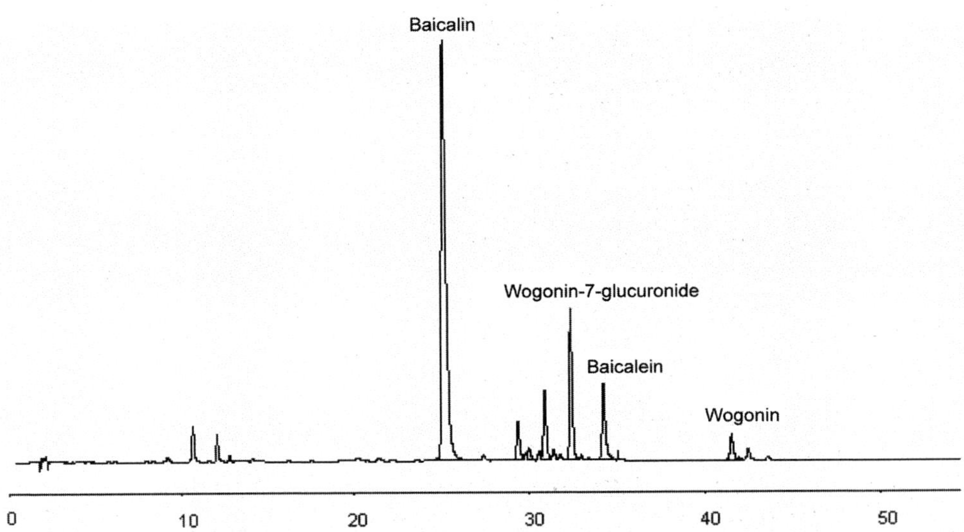

Representative HPLC chromatogram of skullcap run by method 3.

References

1. Suk K, Lee H, Kang SS, et al. Flavonoid baicalein attenuates activation-induced cell death of brain microglia. *J Pharmacol Exp Ther.* 2003;305(2):638–45.
2. Hong T, Jin GB, Cho S, et al. Evaluation of the anti-inflammatory effect of baicalein on dextran sulfate sodium–induced colitis in mice. *Planta Med.* 2002;68(3):268–71.
3. Chung CP, Park JB, Bae KH. Pharmacological effects of methanolic extract from the root of *Scutellaria baicalensis* and its flavonoids on human gingival fibroblast. *Planta Med.* 1995;61(2):150–3.
4. Ishimaru K, Nishikawa K, Omoto T, et al. Two flavone 2′-glucosides from *Scutellaria baicalensis. Phytochemistry.* 1995;40(1):279–81.
5. Miyaichi Y, Imoto Y, Saida H, et al. Studies on the constituents of *Scutellaria* species. (X). On the flavonoid constituents of the leaves of *Scutellaria baicalensis* Georgi. *Shoyakugaku Zasshi.* 1988;42(3):216–9.
6. Takido M, Aimi M, Takahashi S, et al. Constituents in the water extracts of crude drugs. I. Roots of *Scutellaria baicalensis. Yakugaku Zasshi.* 1975;95(1):108–13.
7. Miyaichi Y, Tomimori T. Studies on constituents of *Scutellaria* species. XIX. Lignan glycosides of roots of *Scutellaria baicalensis* Georgi. *Natural Medicines.* 1998;52(1):82–6.
8. Miyaichi Y, Tomimori T. Studies on the constituents of *Scutellaria* species. XVII. Phenol glycosides of the root of *Scutellaria baicalensis* Georgi (2). *Natural Medicines.* 1995;49(3): 350–3.
9. Miyaichi Y, Tomimori T. Constituents of *Scutellaria* species. XVI. On the phenol glycosides of the root of *Scutellaria baicalensis* Georgi. *Natural Medicines.* 1994;48(3):215–8.
10. Ma C, Dai B, Lin R. HPLC quantitative analysis and fingerprint study of 4 flavonoids in *Scutellaria baicalensis. Yaowu Fenxi Zazhi.* 2003;23(2):83–6.
11. Yang L, Liu D, Feng X, et al. Determination of flavone for *Scutellaria baicalensis* from different areas by HPLC. *Zhongguo Zhong Yao Za Zhi.* 2002;27(3):166–70.
12. Liu M, Yang L, Wan Y, et al. Determination of baicalin and wogonoside in 7 species of Scutellariae Radix by RP–HPLC. *Yaowu Fenxi Zazhi.* 2002;22(2):99–102.
13. Zhang YY, Guo YZ, Ageta H, et al. Quantitative analysis of flavonoids in Scutellariae Radix of different sources and seasonal variation by HPLC. *J Chin Pharm Sci.* 1998;7(3):138–41.
14. Xie L, Wang X, Basnet P, et al. Evaluation of variation of acetoside and three major flavonoids in wild and cultivated *Scutellaria baicalensis* roots by micellar electrokinetic chromatography. *Chem Pharm Bull.* 2002;50(7):896–9.
15. Takino Y, Miyahara T, Arichi E, et al. Determination of some flavonoids in Scutellariae Radix by high-performance liquid chromatography. *Chem Pharm Bull.* 1987;35(8):3494–7.
16. Bochorakova H, Paulova H, Slanina J, et al. Main flavonoids in the root of *Scutellaria baicalensis* cultivated in Europe and their comparative antiradical properties. *Phytother Res.* 2003;17(6):640–4.

SOY

Description

Botanical name: *Glycine max* L.

Common name: Soybean

Parts of plant used: Beans

Uses: Prevention of heart disease, possible prevention of osteoporosis and cancer; as a phytoestrogen; beneficial effects on women's health.

Mode of Action

Three groups of compounds—proteins, isoflavones, and saponins—have been found to have beneficial effects on health. Soy proteins lower total cholesterol and low-density lipoproteins, presumably reducing the risk of heart disease. Soy isoflavones are well-known phytoestrogens. Soy saponins also were reported to lower cholesterol and to prevent cancer.

Chemical Markers

Because soy is a valuable crop, its chemical components have been studied extensively. Soybeans are a good source of protein, lipids, sterols, isoflavones, and saponins. It is generally recognized that there are 12 major isoflavones in different soy products, divided into three groups based on the aglycone moiety, namely, daidzein, genistein, and glycitein. In each group, there are four types: isoflavone aglycone, glycoside, 6-acetylglycoside, and 6-malonylglycoside. In nature, 6-malonylglycoside is the most common form, but it is unstable and will decompose with heat. Isoflavone 6-acetylglycoside does not exist in nature; it is produced from 6-malonylglycoside by heat during drying and processing. In addition to these 12 compounds, other isoflavones also were identified in soy products.[1,2]

Soybeans also were reported to contain 5% to 6% soyasaponins.[3] The majority of soyasaponins can be divided into two groups (A and B) based on their aglycone structures. Soyasaponins in group A are bidesmosidic saponins with two glycosylation sites on their aglycones (soyasapogenol A). Group B soyasaponins are monodesmosidic saponins, with only one glycosylation site on the aglycones (soyasapogenols B and E). The genuine soyasaponins of group B in the legume are conjugated with 2,3-dihydro-2,5-dihydroxy-6-methyl-4-pyrone (DDMP), which will degrade to non-DDMP counterparts during heat treatment.[4,5] Currently, the isoflavones and soyasaponins are used as marker compounds for quality control of different soy products.

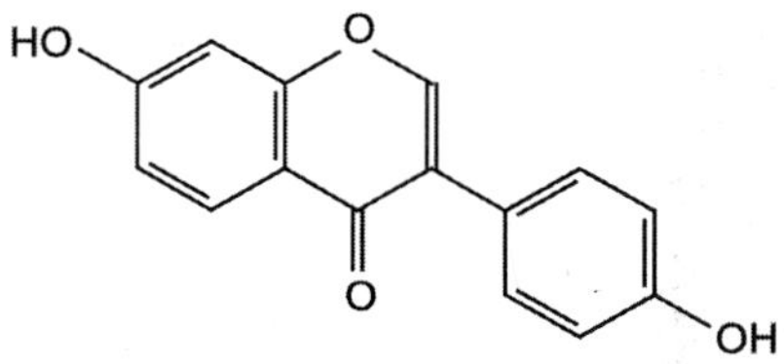

Daidzein

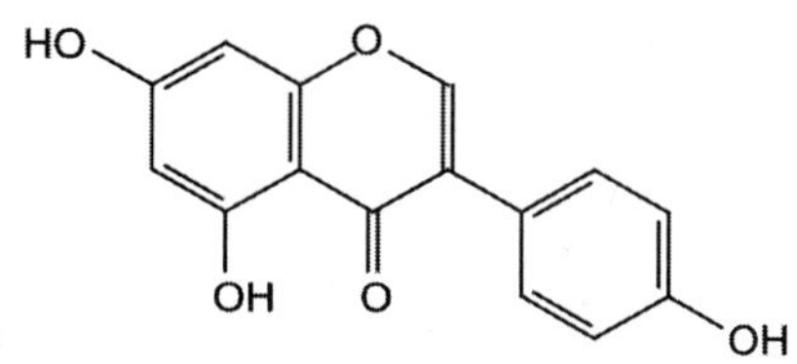

Genistein

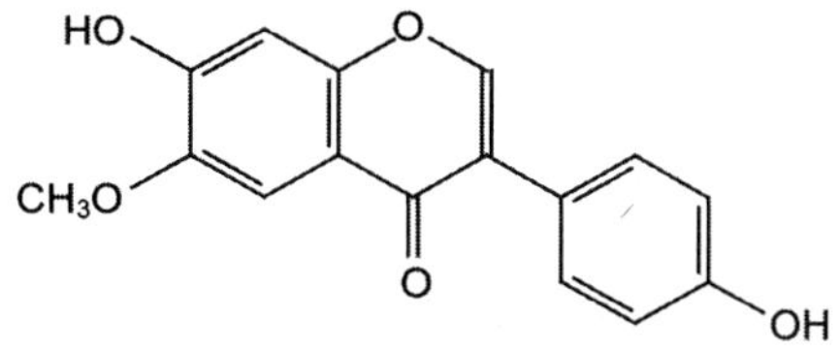

Glycitein

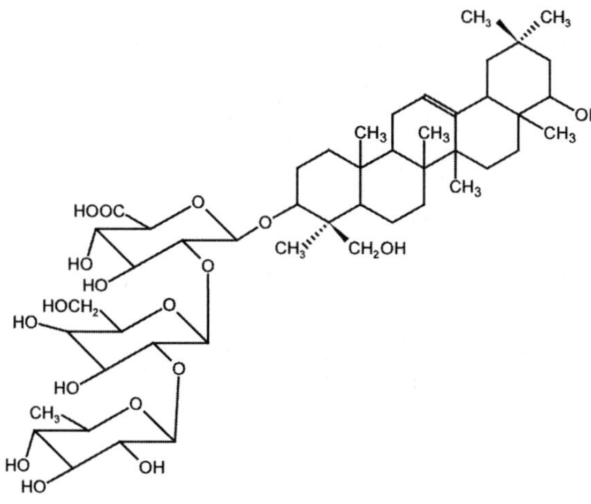

Soyasaponin I

Methods of Analysis

Various methods have been used to analyze the isoflavone content in soy products; the most common method is HPLC coupled with UV and MS detection. HPLC is also the method of choice for analysis of soyasaponins; however, alternate forms of detection such as ELSD and MS should be considered because the poor UV activity of these compounds makes detection with UV very difficult.

Method 1: A method found at www.nsfina.org was used. This method analyzes six isoflavones in various soy products: genistein, genistin, daidzein, daidzin, glycitein, and glycitin.

Sample preparation: For soy flours high in protein, weigh about 1 g into a 50-mL centrifuge tube. Add 40 mL of methanol–water (80:20), cap, and then shake or stir in a 65°C water bath for 2 hours. Cool to room temperature, add 3 mL of 2 N sodium hydroxide, and shake at room temperature for 10 minutes. Add 1 mL of glacial acetic acid, swirl to suspend, and dilute to a 50-mL final volume with methanol–water (80:20). Filter the sample through quantitative-grade filter paper into a 250-mL beaker. Transfer the contents of the beaker to a 50-mL centrifuge tube and centrifuge for 10 minutes at 2000 rpm. Transfer 1 mL of supernate to a 1.5-mL microfuge tube and centrifuge for 10 minutes at 8000–10,000 rpm. Transfer the supernate to HPLC sample vials.

For samples high in isoflavones, weigh about 300 mg of sample into a 50-mL centrifuge tube. Add 40 mL of methanol–water (80:20), cap, and shake or stir in a 65°C water bath for 2 hours. Cool to room temperature, and add 3 mL of 2 N sodium hydroxide, and shake for 10 minutes at room temperature. Add 1 mL of glacial acetic acid and swirl to suspend. Dilute to a 50-mL volume with methanol and centrifuge for 10 minutes at 2000 rpm.

For samples with 40% isoflavones, dilute 1 mL of the supernate to a 10-mL final volume with methanol–water (80:20).

For samples with 20% isoflavones, dilute 2 mL of the supernate to a 10-mL final volume with methanol–water (80:20).

Chromatography

Column: Phenomenex Luna C18(2), 5 µm, 250 × 4.6 mm, or Varian Microsorb MV C18, 5 µm, 250 × 4.6 mm, 100Å.

Mobile phase: Solvent A = water–methanol–10% acetic acid (88:10:2), solvent B = methanol–acetic acid (98:2).

Gradient:

Time (minutes)	%A	%B
0	80	20
2	70	30
10	50	50
16	30	70
16.01	0	100
19	0	100
19.02	80	20
25	80	20

Column temperature: 30°C

Flow rate: 0.8 mL/minute

Injection volume: 10 µL

Detection wavelength: UV at 260 nm

Method 2: The method of Setchell and Cole[6] was used.

Sample preparation: Reflux about 3 to 5 g of powder or liquid sample containing about 0.5 to 2 g of solids with 70 mL of methanol–water (80:20 vol/vol, final ratio) for 1 hour. Cool to room temperature and filter into a 100-mL volumetric flask, wash, and dilute to 100 mL with 80% methanol.

For samples with a high amount of fat, wash out the fats with hexane before sample injection.

Chromatography

Column: C18, 5 μm, 250 × 4.6 mm.

Mobile phase: Solvent A = water (10 mM ammonium acetate and 0.1% trifluoroacetic acid), solvent B = acetonitrile–water (90:10 vol/vol).

Gradient:

Time (minutes)	%A	%B
0	0	100
2	0	100
24	50	50
29	50	50
34	0	100
40	0	100
25	80	20

Detection wavelength: UV at 260 nm

Flow rate: 1.0 mL/minute

Injection volume: 10 μL

Method 3: The unpublished method of Mingfu Wang was used.

Sample preparation: For a soy 40% isoflavone extract, weigh a 50-mg sample into a 50-mL volumetric flask, add about 35 mL of 70% methanol, sonicate for 10 minutes, and shake for 20 minutes. Allow the flask to cool to room temperature and fill to volume with 70% methanol.

Chromatography

Column: Phenomenex Prodigy ODS (3), 5 μm, 150 × 3.2 mm.

Mobile phase: Solvent A = water (0.1% formic acid), solvent B = acetonitrile.

Gradient: 10%B to 35%B in 40 minutes.

Flow rate: 0.8 mL/minute

Injection volume: 10 μL

Detection wavelength: 255 nm

Column temperature: Ambient

Method 4: The method of Dalluge et al.[3] can be used to identify soyasaponins and isoflavones simultaneously in soy products.

Sample preparation: Extract the soy product with 95% aqueous methanol (vol/vol).

Chromatography

Column: Zorbax Eclipse XDB-18, 250 × 4.6 mm.

Mobile phase: Solvent A = water (0.05% trifluoroacetic acid vol/vol), solvent B = acetonitrile (0.05% trifluoroacetic acid vol/vol).

Gradient:

Time (minutes)	%A	%B
0	87	13
25	70	30
35	60	40
47	60	40
55	10	90
65	0	100
70	0	100
72	87	13

Flow rate: 0.5 mL/minute

Injection volume: 25 μL

Detector: MS

Column temperature: Ambient

Method 5: This method of Hu et al.[4] can be used to quantify group B soyasaponins.

Sample preparation: Extract about 4 g of a dried, finely ground soy sample or 0.2 to 1 g of concentrated soy ingredients with 100 mL of 70% aqueous ethanol with stirring for 2.5 hours at room temperature. Filter, then evaporate the extraction solution to dryness at less than 30°C. Dissolve the residue in 10 mL of 80% methanol.

Chromatography

Column: YMC RP-18 or YMC-ODS-AM-303, 5 μm, 250 × 4.6 mm.

Mobile phase: Solvent A = 0.05% trifluoroacetic acid, solvent B = acetonitrile with 0.05% trifluoroacetic acid.

Gradient:

Time (minutes)	%A	%B
0	63	37
12	60	40
37	52	48
38	0	100
40	0	100
45	63	37

Column temperature: 30°C
Flow rate: 1 mL/minute
Injection volume: 50 μL
Detection wavelength: 205 nm

Validation data:
Linearity: Not specified
Accuracy: The percent of recovery for soyasaponin I was between 93.9 and 120.9 for three different products.
Precision: The within-day variation was less than 9.8% and the between-day variation was less than 14.3% for soyasaponin I, II, V, αg, βg, and βa.
Selectivity: Peak identification was determined against standards.
Ruggedness: Not specified
Robustness: Not specified
LOD/LOQ: Not specified

References

1. Hosny M, Rosazza JP. New isoflavone and triterpene glycosides from soybeans. *J Nat Prod*. 2002;65(6):805–13.
2. Gu L, Gu W. Characterisation of soy isoflavones and screening for novel malonyl glycosides using high-performance liquid chromatography-electrospray ionisation-mass spectrometry. *Phytochem Anal*. 2001;12(6):377–82.
3. Dalluge JJ, Eliason E, Frazer S. Simultaneous identification of soyasaponins and isoflavones and quantification of soyasaponin Bb in soy products, using liquid chromatography/electrospray ionization–mass spectrometry. *J Agric Food Chem*. 2003;51(12):3520–4.
4. Hu J, Lee SO, Hendrich S, et al. Quantification of the group B soyasaponins by high-performance liquid chromatography. *J Agric Food Chem*. 2002;50(9):2587–94.
5. Gu L, Tao G, Gu W, et al. Determination of soyasaponins in soy with LC-MS following structural unification by partial alkaline degradation. *J Agric Food Chem*. 2002;50(24):6951–9.
6. Setchell KD, Cole SJ. Variations in isoflavone levels in soy foods and soy protein isolates and issues related to isoflavone databases and food labeling. *J Agric Food Chem*. 2003;51(14):4146–55.

TURMERIC

Description

Botanical names: *Curcuma longa* L.; *Curcuma domestica* Val.

Common names: Common turmeric, haridra, Indian saffron, Jiang-Huang, yellow ginger

Parts of plant used: Rhizomes

Uses: As a food colorant, as an anticancer agent, as an anti-inflammatory agent.

Mode of Action

The health benefits of turmeric have been supported by research, and the bioactivities of curcumins have been studied. Curcumins were found to be antioxidant and anti-inflammatory agents and to suppress tumor initiation, promotion, and metastasis. Curcumins suppress proliferation of a wide variety of tumor cells: they down-regulate transcription factors AP-1, Egr-1, and NF-κB; they down-regulate the expression of COX2, LOX, NOS, MMP-9, TNF, uPA, chemokines, cell surface adhesion mols, and cyclin D1; they down-regulate growth factor receptors; and they inhibit the activity of c-Jun N-terminal kinase, protein tyrosine kinases, and protein serine/threonine kinases.[1,2]

Chemical Markers

Three major curcuminoids (diarylheptane derivatives) are found in turmeric rhizomes: curcumin (the major curcuminoid) and demethoxycurcumin and bisdemethoxycurcumin. The essential oil of turmeric roots has been studied by GC and GC–MS: the rhizome essential oils were highly rich in α- and β-turmerones (40.8%), myrcene (12.6%), 1,8-cineole (7.7%), and p-cymene (3.8%).[3]

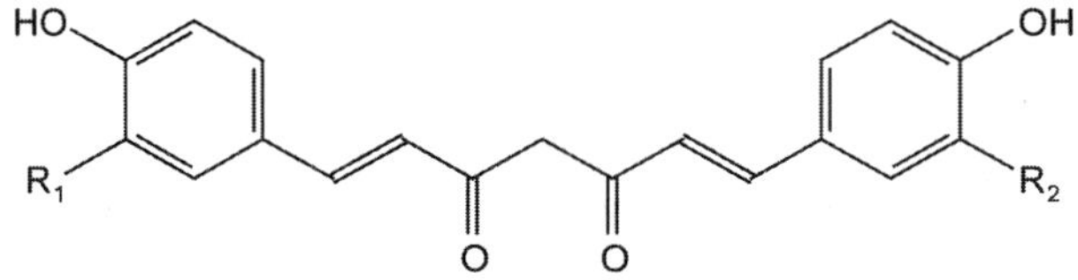

Curcumin: R_1 = OCH_3, R_2 = OCH_3
Demethoxycurcumin: R_1 = OCH_3, R_2 = H
Bisdemethoxycurcumin: R_1 = H, R_2 = H

Methods of Analysis

The curcuminoid content in turmeric powders or powder extracts has been analyzed by various methods including spectrophotometry, TLC, GC–MS, LC–MS, and capillary electrophoresis, but HPLC is the most widely used analytical method.[4–7]

Extraction is key for accurate analysis of curcumins in turmeric. Generally, pure methanol is the selected solvent. The extraction should be handled carefully, avoiding use of strong acids and alkaloids in the extraction and avoiding extra metals in the extraction solvent. The extraction solution should be analyzed as soon as possible because curcumins may degrade.[8]

Method 1: The HPLC method of Jayaprakasha et al.[4] was used.

Sample preparation: Extract turmeric powder (1 g) with 50 mL of hexane using a Soxhlet extractor for 30 minutes. Discard the hexane, and extract the sample with 50 mL of methanol for 2 hours.

Chromatography

Column: Waters µBondapak C18, 300 × 3.9 mm.

Mobile phase: Solvent A = water with 2% acetic acid, solvent B = acetonitrile, solvent C = methanol.

Gradient:

Time (minutes)	%A	%B	%C
0	50	45	5
15	30	65	5
20	50	45	5

Flow rate: 1.0 mL/minute

Injection volume: 10 µL

Detection wavelength: 425 nm

Validation data:

Linearity: 0.0625 to 2.9 mcg for curcumin, demethoxycurcumin, and bisdemethoxycurcumin with correlation coefficients over 0.9844.

Accuracy: Not specified

Precision: Not specified

Selectivity: Peak identification was determined against standards.

Ruggedness: Not specified

Robustness: Not specified

LOD/LOQ: LOQ = 0.05 mcg.

Method 2: The method of Hiserodt et al.[6] was used.

Sample preparation: Sonicate 10 mg of sample in 10 mL of methanol.

Chromatography

Column: Supelcosil LC18, 5 µm, 250 × 4.6 mm.

Mobile phase: Solvent A = water with 1% citric acid (pH adjusted to 3 with sodium hydroxide), solvent B = acetonitrile.

Gradient:

Time (minutes)	%A	%B
0	50	50
10	50	50
40	20	80

Injection volume: 10 µL

Flow rate: 1 mL/minute

Detection wavelength: 423 nm

Validation data:

Linearity: 186 to 929 pg for curcumin, 52 to 258 pg for demethoxycurcumin, and 14 to 71 pg for bisdemethoxycurcumin with correlation coefficients over 0.9989.

Accuracy: Not specified

Precision: 1.68% RSD for curcumin, 0.60% RSD for demethoxycurcumin, and 0.49% RSD for bisdemethoxycurcumin.

Selectivity: Peak identification was determined against standards.

Ruggedness: Not specified

Robustness: Not specified

LOD/LOQ: LOQ = 0.05 mcg.

Method 3: The unpublished method of Mingfu Wang was used.

Sample preparation: Sonicate 500 mg of turmeric powder or 30 mg of curcumin extract in 70 mL of methanol for 30 minutes. Cool to room temperature, and fill to 100 mL with methanol for HPLC analysis.

Chromatography

Column: Phenomenex Prodigy ODS 3, 100Å, 5 µm, 150 × 3.2 mm.

Mobile phase: Solvent A = water with 0.2% phosphoric acid, solvent B = acetonitrile, A/B (60:40) isocratic.

Injection volume: 10 μL
Flow rate: 1 mL/minute
Detection wavelength: 430 nm

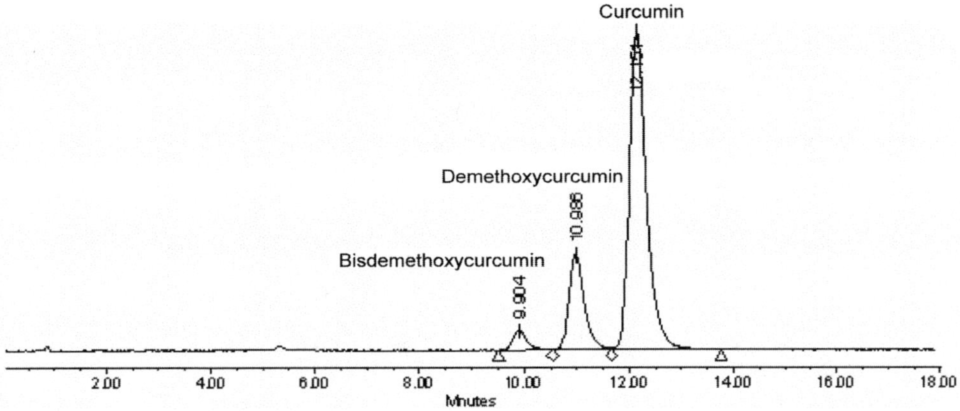

Representative HPLC chromatogram of turmeric extract run by method 3.

References

1. Aggarwal BB, Kumar A, Bharti AC. Anticancer potential of curcumin: preclinical and clinical studies. *Anticancer Res.* 2003;23(1A):363–98.
2. Chauhan DP. Chemotherapeutic potential of curcumin for colorectal cancer. *Curr Pharm Design.* 2002;8(19):1695–706.
3. Bansal RP, Bahl JR, Garg SN, et al. Differential chemical compositions of the essential oils of the shoot organs, rhizomes and rhizoids in the turmeric *Curcuma longa* grown in Indo-Gangetic Plains. *Pharm Biol.* 2002;40(5):384–9.
4. Jayaprakasha GK, Rao LJ, Sakariah KK. Improved HPLC method for the determination of curcumin, demethoxycurcumin, and bisdemethoxycurcumin. *J Agric Food Chem.* 2002;50(13):3668–72.
5. He XG, Lin LZ, Lian LZ, et al. Liquid chromatography–electrospray mass spectrometric analysis of curcuminoids and sesquiterpenoids in turmeric (*Curcuma longa*). *J Chromatogr A.* 1998;818(1):127–32.
6. Hiserodt R, Hartman TG, Ho CT, et al. Characterization of powdered turmeric by liquid chromatography–mass spectrometry and gas chromatography–mass spectrometry. *J Chromatogr A.* 1996;740(1):51–63.
7. Inoue K, Hamasaki S, Yoshimura Y, et al. Validation of LC/electrospray–MS for determination of major curcuminoids in foods. *J Liq Chromatogr Relat Technol.* 2003;26(1):53–62.
8. Cooper TH, Clark JG, Guzinski JA. Analysis of curcuminoids by high-performance liquid chromatography. In: *ACS symposium series 547: food phytochemicals for cancer prevention II.* Washington, DC: American Chemical Society;1994:231–6.

VALERIAN

Description

Botanical name: *Valeriana officinalis* L.

Common names: Garden heliotrope, garden valerian

Parts of plant used: Subterranean parts including the rhizomes and roots.

Uses: Treatment of anxiety, sleep disorders, and insomnia.

Mode of Action

Various clinical trials with valerian have shown positive effects on anxiety, sleep disorders, and mood. Multiple compounds in valerian are believed to be responsible for its activities. These components include iridoids (valepotriates) and their degradation products (baldrinals), sesquiterpenes (valerenic acid, hydroxyvalerenic acid, acetoxyvalerenic acid), essential oil, and even flavonoids (6-methylapigenin, hesperidin). Animal studies have shown that valerenic acid may inhibit enzymes that break down γ-aminobutyric acid (GABA), increasing GABA levels and producing a CNS-depressing effect. In addition, 6-methylapigenin is a benzodiazepine binding site (BDZ-bs) ligand of the GABA receptor.[1,2] These two valerian compounds may work synergistically to produce a sedative effect.

Chemical Markers

Numerous compounds have been identified in valerian. The main ones are iridoids (the iridoid esters valtrate, acevaltrate, isovaltrate, and dihydrovaltrate are very unstable and can be degraded easily by moisture and heat to baldrinal and isopropylbaldrinal), sesquiterpenes (valerenic acid, acetoxyvalerenic acid, hydroxyvalerenic acid), flavonoids (hesperidin, 6-methylapigenin, glycoside derivatives of quercetin, diosmetin, luteolin, apigenin, kaempferol, and acacetin), alkaloids, amino acids, sterols, and tannins.[2–4]

When the essential oil of valerian was studied by GC and GC–MS, the main components were found to be bornyl acetate, spathulenol, valeranone, valerenal, kessyl acetate, and (–)-valerena-4,7(11)-diene.[5] As valerenic acids are bioactive compounds in valerian and are stable, they are used as chemical markers for the quality control of valerian root powders and extracts.

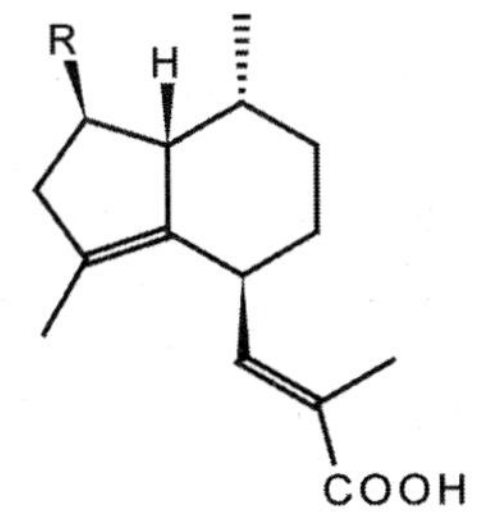

Valerenic acid: R = H
Hydroxyvalerenic acid: R = OH
Acetoxyvalerenic acid: R = OAc

Major valerenic acids found in valerian.

Methods of Analysis

HPLC has been used for the analysis of three types of compounds (valerenic acids, valepotriates, baldrinals) with the valerenic acids used as the quality control standards. Valerenic acids can be extracted easily with 50% ethanol, pure methanol, and 60% acetonitrile through water-bath heating or sonication.

Method 1: The HPLC method of Bokstaller and Schmidt[6] was used for analysis.

Sample preparation: Prepare samples in 50% ethanol.

Chromatography

Column: Merck LiChrospher RP100 C18, 5 µm, 250 × 4.0 mm with a guard column (Merck LiChrospher RP100 C18, 5 µm, 4.0 × 4.0 mm).

Mobile phase: Solvent A = acetonitrile–water (110:690 wt/wt), solvent B = acetonitrile–water (120:180 wt/wt). Both solutions were adjusted to pH 2.8 with 85% phosphoric acid.

Gradient:

Time (minutes)	%A	%B
0	55	45
5	55	45
10	25	75
15	25	75
20	0	100
22	0	100
22.5	55	45

Flow rate: 1.5 mL/minute

Injection volume: 10 µL

Detection wavelength: 225 nm

Validation data: Not available

Method 2: The Chromadex HPLC method was used.

Sample preparation: Weigh about 1 g of 0.8% valerenic acid extract into a 100-mL volumetric flask, add about 50 mL of 60% acetonitrile, and sonicate for 15 minutes. Then cool to room temperature, and dilute to volume with 60% acetonitrile.

Chromatography

Column: Phenomenex Luna C18(2), 5 μm, 150 × 4.6 mm.

Mobile phase: Solvent A = acetonitrile–water–85% phosphoric acid (40:60:0.2), solvent B = acetonitrile–water–85% phosphoric acid (80:20:0.2).

Gradient:

Time (minutes)	%A	%B
0	100	0
20	0	100

Flow rate: 1.5 mL/minute

Injection volume: 10 μL

Detection wavelength: 218 nm

Column temperature: Ambient

Validation data: Not available

Method 3: The unpublished method of Mingfu Wang was used for the HPLC determination of valerenic acids.

Sample preparation: Extract about 200 mg of 0.8% valerenic acid extract with 35 mL of 60% methanol using sonication for 25 minutes. Then cool to room temperature, and dilute to volume with methanol.

Chromatography

Column: Phenomenex Prodigy ODS(3), 5 μm, 150 × 3.2 mm.

Mobile phase: Solvent A = water (adjusted to pH 2.5 with phosphoric acid), solvent B = acetonitrile.

Gradient:

Time (minutes)	%A	%B
0	60	40
8	56	44
22	24	76
27	24	76
27.1	60	40
40	60	40

Flow rate: 0.9 mL/minute
Injection volume: 10 μL
Detection wavelength: 214 nm
Column temperature: Ambient

Method 4: The method of Bos et al.[7] can be used to analyze three types of compounds simultaneously: valerenic acids, valepotriates, and baldrinals.

Sample preparation: Weigh 1.5 g of ground material, add 20 mL of methanol, and reflux in a water bath for 30 minutes. Filter into a 50-mL volumetric flask, add an additional 20 mL of methanol, and reflux for 15 minutes more. Combine the extraction solutions, cool to room temperature, and dilute to volume with methanol.

For capsules, cut capsules, extract the material with three portions of 30 mL of methanol for 5 minutes using sonication. Combine the extraction solutions into a 100-mL volumetric flask, and dilute to volume.

For tablets, grind five tablets together and extract twice with 10 mL of methanol using sonication for 5 minutes. Transfer the extraction solution to a 25-mL volumetric flask, and dilute to volume.

Chromatography

Column: Superspher RP100 C18 (5 μm, LiChroCART 250 × 4.0 mm) with guard column (Merck LiChrospher RP100 C18, 5 μm, LiChroCART 4.0 × 4.0 mm).

Mobile phase: Solvent A = water–acetonitrile (800:156.4 wt/wt), solvent B = water–acetonitrile (200:625.6 wt/wt) (both eluents contain 1 mM phosphoric acid).

Gradient:

Time (minutes)	%A	%B
0	55	45
5	55	45
24	0	100
26	0	100
28	55	45
33	55	45

Flow rate: 1.5 mL/minute

Column temperature: 25°C

Injection volume: 20 μL

Detection wavelength: 256 nm for valtrate, isovaltrate, and acevaltrate; 203 nm for didrovaltrate and isovaleroxyhydroxydidrovaltrate; and 230 and 246 nm for baldrinal and homobaldrinal, respectively.

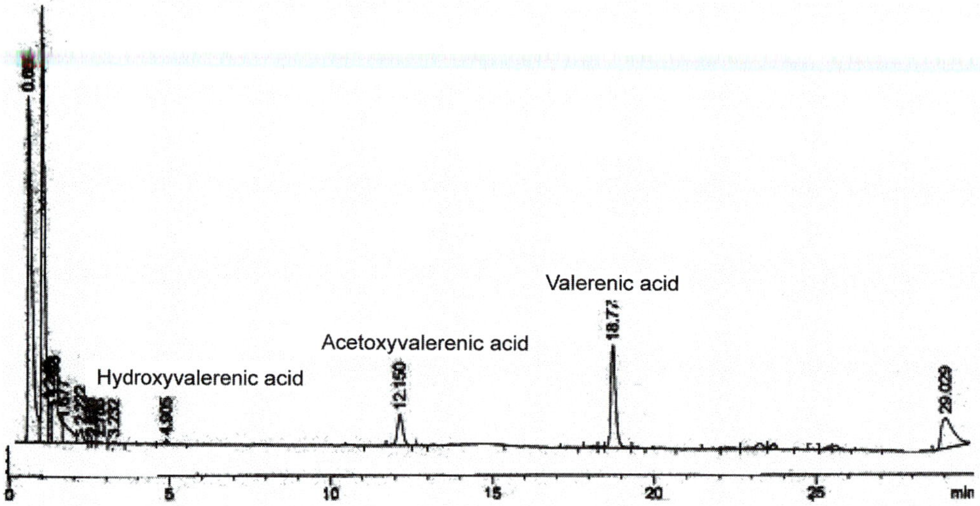

Representative HPLC chromatogram of valerian run by method 3.

References

1. Newell C, Anderson L, Philip J. *Herbal medicine: a guide for health-care professionals.* London: Pharmaceutical Press; 1996:260–2.
2. Marder M, Viola H, Wasowski C, et al. 6-Methylapigenin and hesperidin: new valeriana flavonoids with activity on the CNS. *Pharmacol Biochem Behav.* 2003;75(3):537–45.
3. Bruneton J. *Pharmacognosy, Phytochemistry, Medicinal Plants.* Paris: Lavoisier Publishing; 1995:481–5.
4. Fursa NS. Study of the flavonoid composition of common valerian of the Asian part of the USSR. *Farmatsevtichnii Zhurnal* (Kiev). 1980;3:72–3.
5. Bos R, Hendriks H, Pras N, et al. Essential oil composition of *Valeriana officinalis* ssp. Collins cultivated in Bulgaria. *J Essential Oil Res.* 2000;12(3):313–6.
6. Bokstaller S, Schmidt PC. A comparative study on the content of passionflower flavonoids and sesquiterpenes from valerian root extracts in pharmaceutical preparations by HPLC. *Pharmazie.* 1997;52(7):552–7.
7. Bos R, Woerdenbag HJ, Pras N. Determination of valepotriates. *J Chromatogr A.* 2002;967(1):131–46.

WILLOW BARK

Description

Botanical names: *Salix alba* L. and other species

Common name: White willow bark

Parts of plant used: Inner bark

Uses: For pain relief and fever reduction; as an anti-inflammatory agent.

Mode of Action

Willow bark is known to contain salicin-type compounds that are responsible for its bioactivity. In the human body, salicin decomposes to salicylic acid by oxidation of salicyl alcohol, which is formed upon intestinal hydrolysis of salicin. Salicylic acid is the final bioactive compound.

Chemical Markers

The chemical components of several willow species have been studied thoroughly. The barks were found to contain different amounts of phenolic compounds, depending on the species, the source, the collecting time, and the age of the trees. The identified phenolics include proanthocynidins (monomers, dimers, trimers), flavonoids (rutin, naringenin-7-glucoside, luteolin-7-glucoside, quercitrin, naringenin-5-glucoside, quercetin), glycosides of phenols and phenolic acids (salicin, fragilin, tremuloidin, salicortin, tremulacin, populin).[1,2] Currently, salicin is used as a marker compound for quality control of willow bark extract, especially white willow bark extract.

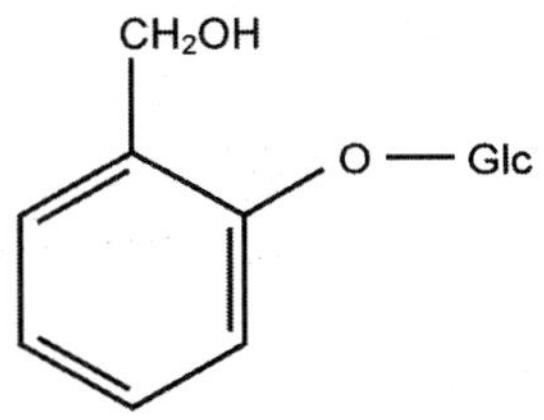

Salicin

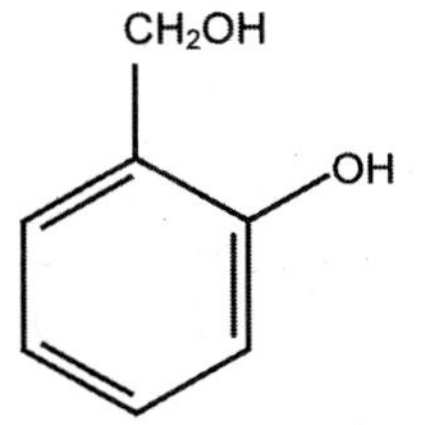

Salicyl alcohol

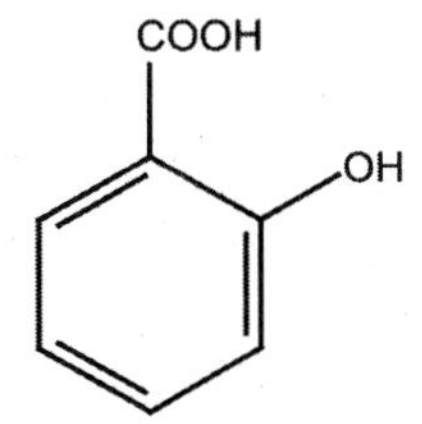

Salicylic acid

Methods of Analysis

Although willow bark has been known for its anti-inflammatory activity for a long time, only a few analytical methods have been applied to analyze the phenolic compounds in it. Currently, HPLC is the most widely used method for analysis of salicin in willow bark extract.

Method 1: The HPLC method of Meier et al.[3] was used.

Sample preparation: Extract 200 to 500 mg of dried material in a clipping homogenisator with 25 mL of methanol, then with 40 mL of methanol, and then with 20 mL of methanol. Evaporate the solution to dryness at less than 40°C. Dissolve the residue in 10 mL of methanol–water (7:2).

Chromatography

Column: Spherisorb ODS (2), 5 μm, 100 × 4 mm.

Mobile phase: Solvent A = water–tetrahydrofuran–phosphoric acid (97.7:1.8:0.5), solvent B = methanol.

Gradient:

Time (minutes)	%A	%B
0	100	0
5	100	0
10	85	15
20	70	30
30	65	35
40	50	50
45	50	50

Flow rate: 1 mL/minute

Injection volume: 10 μL

Detection wavelength: 270 nm

Validation data: Not available

Method 2: In the method of Luo et al.,[4] the salicins are first converted to salicyl alcohol by enzymes and then analyzed by HPLC.

Sample preparation: Extract 1 g of powdered sample with 20 mL of extraction buffer (0.01 M aqueous potassium phosphate containing 0.02% sodium dodecyl sulfate, final pH 5.0) in an 80°C water bath for 30 minutes. Centrifuge for 10 minutes at 2000 × g and dilute 0.5 mL of the supernate to 10 mL with extraction buffer. Pipette 1 mL of diluted extract into a 10-mL test tube and add 1 mL of beta-glucosidase solution (2 mg/mL). Incubate the mixture at 37°C for 40 minutes.

Chromatography

Column: Phenomenex Prodigy ODS-3, 5 μm, 250 × 4.6 mm.

Mobile phase: Solvent A = water (0.02 M KH_2PO_4 with 0.014% tetrabutylammonium hydrogen sulfate), solvent B = acetonitrile; isocratic 84%A and 16%B.

Injection volume: 100 μL

Detection: Fluorescence detector with λ_{ex} = 275 nm and λ_{em} = 300 nm for the first 12 minutes, and then switch to λ_{ex} = 295 nm and λ_{em} = 400 nm.

Flow rate: 1 mL/minute for the first 12 minutes, then increase to 1.5 mL/minute.

Validation data:

Linearity: 8 to 800 mcg/g for salicin and 2 to 160 mcg/g for salicylic acid.

Accuracy: More than 96% recovery with a correlation coefficient of 0.9998 for salicin and more than 89% recovery with a correlation coefficient of 0.9999 for salicylic acid; three types of willow bark were tested.

Precision: Not specified

Selectivity: Peak identification was determined against standards.

Ruggedness: Not specified

Robustness: Not specified

LOD/LOQ: LODs = 4 mcg/g for salicin and 0.05 mcg/g for salicylic acid; LOQs = 20 and 1 mcg/g for salicin and salicylic acid, respectively.

Method 3: The unpublished method of Mingfu Wang was used.

Sample preparation: Weigh the appropriate amount of material (150 mg for 15% white willow extract) into a 50-mL volumetric flask. Add about 35 mL of 20% methanol and sonicate for 20 minutes and shake for 20 minutes. Allow the flask to cool to room temperature and fill to volume with 20% methanol.

Chromatography

Column: Phenomenex Luna C18(2), 5 μm, 250 × 4.6 mm.

Mobile phase: Solvent A = 1% acetic acid solution, solvent B = acetonitrile.

Gradient: 8%B to 32%B in 20 minutes.

Flow rate: 0.8 mL/minute

Injection volume: 10 μL

Detection wavelength: 271 nm

References

1. Balbaa SI, Khafagy SM, Haggag MY, et al. Phytochemical study of certain *Salix* species cultivated in Egypt. *Egypt J Pharm Sci.* 1979;20(1–4):153–64.
2. Bruneton J. *Pharmacognosy, Phytochemistry, Medicinal Plants.* Paris: Lavoisier Publishing; 1995:222–3.

3. Meier B, Julkunen-Tiitto R, Tahvanainen J, et al. Comparative high-performance liquid chromatographic determination of phenolic glucosides in Salicaceae species. *J Chromatogr A*. 1988;442:175–86.
4. Luo W, Ang CY, Schmitt T, et al. Determination of salicin and related compounds in botanical dietary supplements by liquid chromatography with fluorescence detection. *J AOAC Int*. 1998;81:757–62.

Index of Subjects in Introductory Material

Index of Botanical & Common Names

O

P

R

S

T

U

V

W

Y

Z

Index of Dietary Supplements by Use

Index of Chemical Markers

C

D

E

F

G

H

I

K